First Aid for Hill Walkers and Climbers

Stewart Hulse was born in Bury, Lancashire, in 1935, and educated at St Chad's Junior School and East Ward Secondary Modern School. After leaving school he gained his City and Guilds certificate in engineering. After National Service in the REME, he joined Bury Ambulance Service, and gained the St John Ambulance certificate for advanced first aid. In 1964 Mr Hulse and his wife, Joan, moved to the Lake District. He was a founder member of the Ambleside Fell Rescue Team, which later amalgamated with the Langdale Rescue Team to become the Langdale/Ambleside Mountain Rescue Team, and is at present the busiest rescue team in Great Britain, with an average of nearly forty call-outs a year. Mr Hulse is Incidents Officer for the Team and also lectures on mountain safety to schools and colleges in the North of England. In addition, Mr Hulse works as maintenance engineer for South Lakeland District Council and is actively involved with community affairs in Ambleside. Mr Hulse has two children, Caroline and David.

Jane Renouf was born in Oxford in 1949, and attended Notre Dame Junior School, and the Convent of St Clotilde, Lechlade. After leaving school, she gained a joint honours degree in English and Philosophy at Kent University, and after graduating in 1970, joined the staff of the *Croydon Advertiser* as a junior reporter. After a few years, she and her husband, Paul, decided to give up city life and office jobs in favour of a more peaceful, rural life in the Lake District. They moved to Ambleside and bought a guest house, which they run together, and Mrs Renouf also works as a freelance district reporter for the *Westmorland Gazette*.

Jane Renouf and
Stewart Hulse

First Aid for Hill Walkers and Climbers

Illustrations by Bryan Marsh
Medical Adviser: Dr David Earnshaw, M.B., CH.B.

ISBN 0 902363 45 X

First published in Penguin Books 1978
New edition published 1982 by Cicerone Press
Reprinted 1984, 1989

CICERONE PRESS,

MILNTHORPE, CUMBRIA

CONTENTS

Preface 8
Acknowledgements 10

INTRODUCTION
Weather 14; Terrain 16; Equipment 17;
The First-Aid Kit 19

PART ONE: AN ACCIDENT HAS HAPPENED
Emergency Action Quick Reference 25; Immediate
Action 27; The Safety of the Victim 27; The Importance
of Shelter 28; Should I Give a Drink? 30; The
Removal of Clothing 31; How Serious Are the
Injuries? 33; Keeping a Record 38; Mystery
Illnesses 38; Deciding Whether to Send for Help 39

PART TWO: GOING FOR HELP
Emergency Action Quick Reference 43; Parties of
Three or More 44; Parties of Two 45; Walking or
Climbing Alone 47; Rescue Posts and Stretcher Boxes 47

PART THREE: FIRST-AID PRACTICE
ARTIFICIAL RESUSCITATION 54
    General 55
    Mouth-to-Mouth Assisted Breathing 59
    Cardiac Compression 62
ASTHMA 66
BITES, see INSECT STINGS AND BITES 144
BLEEDING 68
    General 68

From the Scalp   73
From the Ear   74
From the Nose   74
From the Palm   75
From a Varicose Vein   76
From a Miscarriage   77
BLISTERS   77
BROKEN BONES, see FRACTURES   103
BURNS   80
CHEST INJURY   84
CRAMP   86
DIABETES   88
   General   88
   Insulin Reaction   89
   Diabetic Coma   91
DROWNING   93
EXPOSURE, see HYPOTHERMIA   134
FATIGUE   95
FITS AND SEIZURES   97
FOOD POISONING   99
FOREIGN OBJECTS IN THE EYE   100
FRACTURES   103
   General   103
   Immobilization   107
   Of the Skull   108
   Of the Ribs   109
   Of the Shoulders, Collar Bone, Arms and Wrists   110
   Of the Pelvis   113
   Of the Thigh   115
   Of the Lower Leg and Ankle   119
   Of the Foot   120
   Of the Spine, see SPINAL INJURY   162
FROSTNIP AND FROSTBITE   121
HEAD INJURIES   124
HEART ATTACK   128
HEATSTROKE   131
HYPOTHERMIA   134
INSECT STINGS AND BITES   144

LIGHTNING 149
MISCARRIAGE, see BLEEDING 77
NOSEBLEED, see BLEEDING 74
PERIOD PAINS 152
SHOCK 153
SNAKE BITES 157
SNOWBLINDNESS 161
SPINAL INJURIES 162
STINGS, see INSECT STINGS AND BITES 144
SUNSTROKE 164
VARICOSE VEINS, see BLEEDING 76
VERTIGO 165

Bibliography 167

PREFACE

This book has been written for those who have very little or no knowledge of first aid. Its aim is to reduce the amount of misguided and dangerous first-aid practice which is occurring at present among hill walkers and climbers. It is in no way intended to replace the first-aid courses already being run by such bodies as the Red Cross and the St John Ambulance Brigade, which provide a far more extensive training and can be applied far more widely. Similarly, while certain aspects of basic preparation for the hills have been included, they are by no means comprehensive and are no substitute for a specialized work on hillcraft.

We have described how to cope with the emergencies most likely to be encountered, drawing on the experience of rescue team members themselves, and walkers and climbers all over Britain, as well as doctors particularly familiar with mountain accidents. We have concentrated on the specific dangers of the mountains so that an interest and a basic working competence in first aid can be acquired without distracting the reader with accidents which are unlikely to occur.

The book will easily fit in your pocket or rucksack every time you go on the hills, but if it is to be useful in an emergency it is essential that you should read it before you start off. For ease of reference, Part Three, which deals with particular accidents and illnesses, is arranged alphabetically.

If you follow the suggestions contained in this book, you will already have acquired a first-aid kit suitable for the hills, and you will know how to use it. You will be prevented from doing the wrong thing in a mountain emergency, and you will be able to judge when the best first aid lies in doing nothing. Prevention is always better than cure; but accidents can still happen however well prepared you may be.

Of course, there will be people who read this book and yet fail to equip themselves adequately. For these people, there may still be a chance to do the right thing, and the book will tell you what limited help you may still be able to give without a proper kit.

Don't feel that you are being over-cautious or over-anxious by carrying the book in your rucksack. Remember the words of one of the country's most experienced climbers, Peter Greenall, who said: 'Never go on the mountains without a degree of cowardice. If you overcome this cowardice, that is the time when you will be putting your life at risk.'

ACKNOWLEDGEMENTS

The authors wish to express their thanks to the following individuals who gave advice, help or constructive criticism in the production of this book. The appearance of their names does not constitute an endorsement of its contents. Frank Davies; Peter Greenall; Irvine Hunt; Dr Geoffrey Lancaster; Bryan Marsh; Eric Penman; Paul Renouf; Bryan Stilling; Cynthia Thompson and Herbert Hartley; and to the following for their help with illustrations: Dave Brown; Barry Knowles; Brian Morgan; Tom Redfern; Tony Richards; Norman Walker.

INTRODUCTION

Mountaineering and hill-walking are among the fastest-growing leisure activities. Interest in more active holiday pursuits has been growing; holidays are becoming more frequent for many people and improvements in communication are bringing mountainous areas within easier reach of city populations. Every year, thousands of people are discovering for the first time the relative ease with which some of the highest and wildest regions can be explored and how the challenge and sense of personal achievement missing from their daily lives can be found by pitting themselves physically and mentally against remote landscapes and the elements. Trends in education have also increased the numbers of children and young people using the hills, for outdoor activities have become an accepted part of school curricula and various organizations and award schemes include hill-walking as part of their tests of personal endurance.

Injuries and deaths in the United Kingdom reported to the Mountain Rescue Committee, 1976

(Figures in brackets indicate fatalities)

	Total	Injured	Fatal	Climbing	Walking	Caving	Natural Causes
WALES	48	43	5	21(3)	27(2)	—	—
PENNINES	50	48	2	17	23(1)	10(1)	1
LAKES	118	105	13	28(7)	90(6)	—	3(3)
SCOTLAND	61	49	12	25(5)	36(7)	—	2
OTHER AREAS	3	—	3	3(3)	—	—	—
TOTAL	280	245	35	94(18)	176(16)	10(1)	6(3)

Predictably, the increased use of the hills has led to a large increase in the number of deaths and reported accidents. The table shows the figures for 1976, and many more unreported incidents involving minor injuries must have occurred. The circumstances of many of these indicate that people are not taking the mountains seriously enough. It is not the main purpose of this book to encourage a greater respect for the mountains, although many accidents are caused through ignorance, poor preparation, lack of basic equipment and general carelessness and could therefore have been avoided. Anyone planning a mountain walk or climb should have some knowledge of such essentials as route-finding, use of compass, suitable equipment and weather conditions.

Why is first aid on the hills so different from ordinary first aid? It is because of the length of time which so often elapses before experienced medical help can reach the victim of a mountain accident. Hills are remote and peaceful. But it is this remoteness, so tempting and desirable to many, which can often leave a victim in quite desperate isolation when help is urgently needed. By getting away from it all, you have also left behind you the normal network of available help. In our homes, workplaces and familiar towns and roads, we have become accustomed to take the services of police, ambulancemen, doctors and hospitals for granted. We are normally never out of range of a telephone and we have come to expect the emergency services to arrive within minutes. Obviously such service cannot be available in remote country.

The height alone of an area is not necessarily a guide to the time it may take for help to arrive. Roads pass over, or near, some of the highest regions, while vast acres of lower uplands may be miles from the nearest motorist or telephone. Roads run on each side of the Brecon Beacons in Wales, for example, making it fairly simple for help to reach this area of very rugged hills; yet in the Cheviot Hills of north-east England, where the land is gentler and less precipitous, you can still walk a distance of twenty-five miles without so much as crossing a cart track. The popularity of particular hills can be a considerable factor in ease of communication; for example, the Peak District National Park, with its 542 square miles of elevated moorland plateaux, potholes, caves and crags, lies within seventy miles of half the total population of Britain. Although the region is fairly remote from road traffic, it is a popular area of recreation for many town dwellers. Even if you are miles from the nearest road, you probably won't be so far away from other walkers, certainly in the summer months.

Nevertheless, it is more often a matter of several hours rather than minutes before professional help can gain access to the scene of a mountain accident. For this reason, mountain first aid plays a vital role in saving lives and preventing further complications. The first-aider in the street may need to do nothing more demanding than give comfort until help arrives. In the hills the first-aider may have the survival of the victim entirely in his own hands.

Yet, despite the obvious importance of first-aid knowledge for anybody using the mountains, rescue teams in Britain are finding that not only do some people know nothing at all about first aid, but often those who think they know what to do make matters very much worse by incorrect action. Doing the wrong thing can have worse results than doing nothing at all. There is no shortage of horror stories to illustrate these points. Victims have bled to death because companions failed to take the most simple common-sense steps to control bleeding, while others have died of cold, spurred on to 'keep walking at all costs' by friends who knew no better.

The plain fact is that the wrong action can kill. Sometimes it kills outright. At other times, when injuries are not in themselves too serious, a wrong action can set in motion a chain of events which can end in death. Two examples of this occurred recently in the Lake District. A middle-aged woman in an organized walking party slipped and punctured a varicose vein in her leg while enjoying a fairly simple walk. She almost died from loss of blood in the three hours that it took for a rescue team to reach her, because none of her companions had successfully discovered how to control the bleeding. It probably would have required no more than direct pressure on the raised leg with a pad of thick material. It sounds simple, but would you have known what to do? In another incident, a school teacher in charge of a walking party of children nearly let one of his pupils die after tying a tight tourniquet around the child's cut leg and leaving it for two hours – he thought this was the right thing to do. Quick action on the part of the rescuer saved the child's life – and his legs – but other victims have not always been so fortunate.

Weather

It may seem unnecessarily gloomy to dwell in such detail on the possibility of mishaps on the hills, but walking and climbing in Britain involve certain dangers which few people know about. The first is the severity of weather conditions. It is no exaggeration to say that winter conditions in Britain can compare with anything that a mountaineer would be likely to encounter in the Alps or even the Himalayas. Seasoned Alpine climbers, and even veterans of Everest, have described setting out in perfect weather in winter in the Cairngorms only to find themselves fighting for their lives against a sudden blizzard. The best-equipped and most experienced have lived to tell the tale, but sadly others hit by these unpredictable and dramatic weather changes have lost their lives.

But it isn't just the wildest, highest and most isolated areas where accidents occur. Britain is a land of contrasting climatic conditions, with temperatures ranging from 32° Centigrade (90° Farenheit) in summer to −20°C (−4°F) in a cold winter. Weather can vary enormously; for example, just twenty miles from the palm trees of the mild south-west coast, where snow falls an average of less than five days in any one year, there is the popular Dartmoor National Park, where snow often lies for twenty days or more. Extreme conditions have claimed several victims here, although only one hill is over 2,000 feet. Weather also behaves in very strange ways; cold air in winter can flow downhill and create a frost hollow in what might appear to be an ideal valley for shelter.

Low temperatures alone, however, do not often cause death. A combination of rain and chill winds can cause hypothermia, or exposure (as a later section will explain in detail). Such conditions can be found on Dartmoor, the Malverns, Mendips, Peaks or Pennines and will kill just as easily as a blizzard on the higher altitudes of the Cairngorms or Scafell.

Rainfall is of particular interest and concern to anyone walking or climbing; rainy conditions can mean poor visibility, wet and slippery rock, sodden footpaths and wet gear, and, when combined with strong winds, a wind chill factor which can cause extreme cold. It is even more important to consider rainfall figures in Britain in the light of the enormous contrasts between the dry east and wet west halves of the country – some of the wettest areas of the western half are also the most popular hills and mountains for walkers and climbers. According to records kept by the Meteorological Office, the wettest place on average anywhere in the British Isles is Styhead in the Lake District; and rainfall over the Lakes on average is approximately ten times higher than that over East Anglia. Few walkers and climbers of any experience will have escaped the vagaries of the west-coast climate and extremes of rainfall.

For although, as a general rule, the west is much wetter than the east, there can also be very large variations from month to month and year to year in the west itself. These contrasts can best be seen in rainfall figures from the Meteorological Office.

For example, Styhead (height 326 metres, 1,069 feet) has a monthly average for January of 435 mm (17 ins.), but in January 1975 the total rainfall was 840·7 mm (33 ins.). The annual average rainfall for Styhead, according to figures collected between 1941 and 1970, is 4,306 mm (169 ins.).

At Cribgoch, in the popular walking and climbing country of North Wales (height 713 metres, 2,339 feet), the monthly average for January is 462 mm (18 ins.), but in the wet January of 1975 a total of 858·5 mm (33 ins.) was recorded. The annual average for Cribgoch (1941–70) is 4,282 mm (168 ins.).

The western coastal area of Scotland also provides similar extremes of rainfall. At Allt Mhoille in Argyllshire (height 503 metres, 1,650 feet) the monthly average for December is 438 mm (17 ins.), but in December 1974 the rainfall amounted to 800 mm (31 ins.). The annual average for Allt Mhoille is 3,714 mm (146 ins.).

Terrain

Weather is not the only common cause of mishaps on the hills. Mountainous terrain is in itself a difficult environment, with its own dangers. The going can be rough and you can easily lose a footing, slip, fall or even be struck by a falling rock. Risks are present in mountainous country which do not exist elsewhere, and they are often outside the normal expectations of the walker. In addition, the physical strain involved in walking or climbing can bring about fatigue which increases the chance of falling victim to the unfamiliar terrain.

Given such conditions, it is to be expected that injuries, when they occur in the hills, can be extremely severe and require good first-aid abilities. Although there are dozens of minor accidents every year involving easily treated injuries, a high proportion of very serious injuries are among the total number of casualties. These are mainly the result of long falls down rock faces, scree slopes or steep hillsides and include injuries such as the severing of arms and legs and even decapitation. Sudden illness can be equally serious and dramatic on the hills, especially to those unused to strenuous activity. The exertion required to meet the challenges of walking and climbing places an enormous strain on their bodies.

Equipment

If you don't know what basic equipment you need as a walker or climber, you don't yet know enough about the mountains to be setting out at all. This can be remedied either by reading some of the pamphlets issued about use of the hills, or by a visit to your local library or bookshop to find a book on hillcraft, or by calling in at information centres run by bodies such as the National Trust or the National Parks. However, it is not enough to draw up a shopping list of essential items such as maps and compass, boots and anorak; that is just the start. Before venturing out, you must learn how to use your equipment. Practise with the compass and a map in an area you know – and then remember that you will be using them in unfamiliar country, possibly in violent weather conditions and in limited visibility. Can you interpret an Ordnance Survey map? Could you do it in a Force-Nine gale with hailstones stinging your face? Many a map has ended its useful life prematurely at the bottom of a hill, snatched from the hands of its user by a gust of wind. Would you know what to do then? Try to visualize the worst possible conditions you are likely to encounter.

Personal comfort is equally important. You should have a good pair of strong, waterproof boots, and you will be wise to take the trouble to wear them in before subjecting your feet to the rigours of a day on the hills in stiff new boots. Blisters account for the greatest of minor miseries afflicting walkers on the hills. They may seem trivial, but they certainly do not feel trivial. They may rob you of important concentration, and can contribute to exhaustion in adverse conditions. Another minor, but important, preparation for any excursion into the hills is to ensure that toenails are cut. Failure to do so can lead to bloodied toes and to considerable discomfort, and is an additional contributory cause of blisters. Such minor inconveniences could lay the foundations to a major mishap.

Besides map, compass, boots and adequately warm and

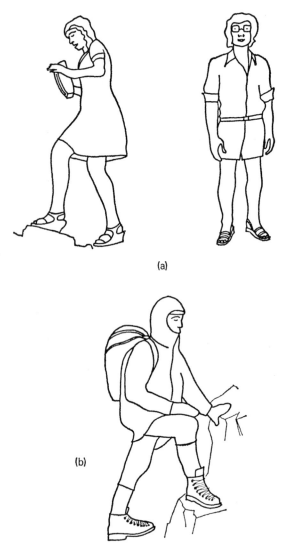

Fig. 1. Clothing and footwear: (a) Incorrect; (b) Correct.

waterproof clothing, you should always carry a spare sweater, a supply of food, including sweets or Mintcake with energy-producing glucose, a torch in case you become benighted on the hills, and a whistle to attract attention if you are alone and need help. If it is winter, you should also be carrying a polythene survival bag; this is a very simple piece of equipment, but one which has saved many lives threatened by hypothermia.

The First-Aid Kit

Many years of first-aid experience on the hills by the rescuers who have helped in producing this book have enabled them to draw up a list of twelve items most commonly needed in mountain first aid. They are inexpensive, and can be bought from any chemist to make a good basic first-aid kit. You may think of other things to add to it, but these versatile items are all that you will need to put the instructions in this book into practice.

Each kit is sufficient for one person. If you are walking in a party of two, ideally you should both have your separate kits. If you are walking in a group, common sense will tell you that not all the members of the party will need to carry a kit. Remember, however, that the party may become accidentally separated or may agree to split up, and in this event make sure that each small group has a couple of kits between them.

The kit should consist of the following:

FOUR TRIANGULAR BANDAGES
FOUR STERILE WOUND DRESSINGS (2 medium and 2 large)
ONE ROLL OF ZINC OXIDE STICKING PLASTER (1–1½ ins. wide)
ONE PAIR OF ROUND-NOSED SCISSORS
ONE 3-INS. CREPE BANDAGE
ONE TIN OF ASSORTED STRETCH-FABRIC PLASTERS

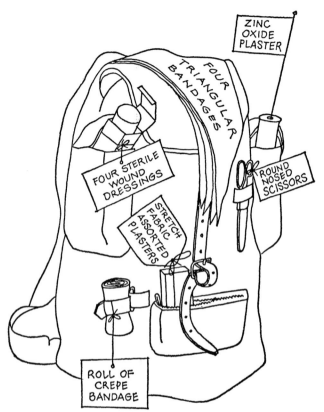

Fig. 2. Twelve items of first-aid equipment.

Triangular Bandages

These triangular pieces of material can be folded in a variety of ways (Figure 3). They can be put to a number of uses: to immobilize or support fractured limbs; to hold a dressing over a wound in an awkward part of the body (though the crepe bandage is usually better for this); and to form extra padding to control cases of severe bleeding. These uses are

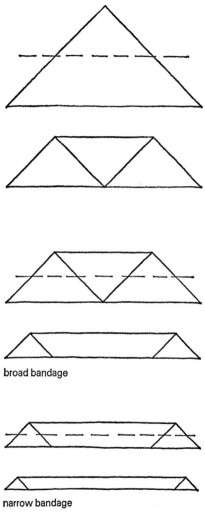

broad bandage

narrow bandage

Fig. 3. How to fold a triangular bandage.

all explained in the appropriate sections. Make sure you have a couple of large safety-pins in the kit to help hold a sling in position more firmly if necessary, or to pin a crepe bandage in place.

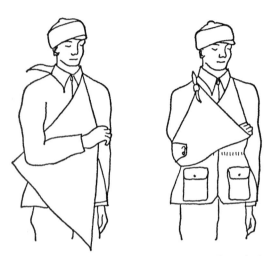

Fig. 4. Supporting injured right arm using a triangular bandage as a sling.

Sterile Dressings

These pads attached to gauze bandages can be used to help stop bleeding, by placing them with direct pressure over wounds and cuts; to help in cases of sprains and bruises, by soaking them in cold water and applying to the injured area as a cold compress and support; to form extra padding to control bleeding; or to fill out a hollow for greater comfort when bandaging an awkwardly situated wound.

Small dressings can be made from sterile dressings by cutting the bandage ends into strips, folding them into a neat pad, and sticking that to a length of sticking plaster. These little dressings are especially useful when a bulkier pad round the victim's foot or ankle would make the boot uncomfortable.

Sticking Plaster or Tape

This very useful item should either be 2·5 cm (1 in.) or 3·75 cm (1½ ins.) wide. You can use the roll both in first aid and for emergency repairs to almost anything. (If you do use it for repairs, make sure you don't run out before an emergency.)

We have already described how the plaster can be used to make your own small dressings, and it is especially useful to secure dressings to the skin when the injured part will continue to be used after the accident.

Never, never put sticking plaster or tape over an open wound without first placing a dressing directly over it. If you do, the sticky backing will adhere to the raw, broken flesh, and will be very painful and difficult to remove. This applies to any damaged skin, and it is just as harmful to place sticky tape directly over a burn or blister. It seems rather an obvious point to stress, but thoughtless first-aiders make this mistake very frequently.

Scissors

Scissors should have round, blunt ends, as pointed ends might inflict injury in the event of a fall. Make sure they are sharp, as they may be required to cut clothing.

The method of carrying and packing your first-aid kit is a matter of personal choice, and some may prefer to have it together rather than spread out in pockets and different parts of a rucksack, as illustrated. If packed together use a polythene bag in which the kit can be kept dry.

It is not necessary to carry much more in the way of first-aid items. Some people may want to include extra things, but the kit should be kept as simple as possible. It is always wise to include some tablets for pain relief like

Panadol or Disprin, and guidance will be given later when these should not be given to casualties. One or two indigestion tablets would also not be amiss, and in summer, salt tablets are a good idea.

Personal medications should never be forgotten, and supplies adequate for two or three days are a wise precaution in case of delay on your trip. Make sure you carry on you a card describing your complaint, and a written list of the medications you are taking, their quantity, strength and frequency. The name and address of your doctor and the name of your next of kin should be given.

AN ACCIDENT HAS HAPPENED

Emergency Action Quick Reference

Urgent action is necessary in the following cases because there is danger of immediate death:

BREATHING STOP
HEART STOP
SEVERE EXTERNAL BLEEDING
HEAD INJURY
SPINAL INJURY
CHEST INJURY

Order of Action

When any of the above injuries has obviously occurred DON'T PANIC. Try to remain cool and calm, but act quickly. DON'T MOVE the victim, especially in the case of spinal injury, unless absolutely necessary to prevent further injury, or unless first aid is impossible without moving him. To move a victim of such injuries can kill or cripple.

If the victim is still breathing and the injuries are not immediately obvious, but because of the nature of the incident, for example, a long fall, you have reason to suspect severe damage, proceed as follows:

EXAMINE at once for SEVERE BLEEDING and STOP IT.

EXAMINE and DIAGNOSE ANY OTHER IN-
JURY (see pages 33–8).
BEGIN FIRST AID, if you can, moving the victim
ONLY if injuries permit and the victim is conscious.

If breathing has stopped, CHECK AIRWAY (page 58),
if necessary start assisted breathing AT ONCE (pages
59–61).
If HEART has stopped, start cardiac compression AT
ONCE (pages 62–6).
If SEVERE EXTERNAL BLEEDING is apparent,
STOP IT AT ONCE (page 68).
For HEAD injury see page 124.
For SPINAL injury see page 162.
For CHEST injury see page 84.

If the victim is conscious, give comfort and reassurance to
reduce shock.
     REMAIN ALERT constantly to the possibility of
stoppage of heart or breathing.
     Decide whether assistance is required and if so send for
help (see pages 39–49).
     Give shelter, warmth and comfort until recovery or until
help arrives.
     Give food or drink ONLY IF ADVISABLE accord-
ing to the nature of the injury or illness. (See instructions
for specific conditions.)

──────────────────────────────────

The foregoing is a guide for quick reference in emergencies.
What follows is a more detailed guide to procedure in the
event of an accident and should be read when any initial
life-saving action has been completed. You *must* read it at
leisure before setting foot on the hills in order to familiarize
yourself with it before the need to use it arises.
     First of all, don't let your own shocked reaction to what
has happened make you the next victim. Don't rush and

don't panic. If you lose control, your first hurried actions could be wrong and careless.

Immediate Action

Before you do anything else, check that the victim is alive and breathing without obstruction. If he is not, and if there is any chance of saving his life, you will have to start artificial resuscitation without delay (see page 54). If you should ever need to give the 'kiss of life' or try to start a heart beating again, you will need plenty of good luck if you have not read that particular section in advance and have a clear understanding of what to do. If you have no idea at all and have to turn to the relevant pages and try to follow the instructions, it may well be too late to save a life.

If things don't seem as urgent as this and the victim is alive and breathing, begin by assessing the extent of the injuries. Refer to page 33 for methods of examination and diagnosis. You must then decide whether you require assistance from a rescue organization. If you are in doubt, refer to page 39. If you decide assistance is required, follow the guidelines set out on page 43. Once you have done this, you can start giving practical help and comfort to the victim. If you are dealing with a conscious casualty, the first thing to give him is confidence. Stay calm and unhurried, and talk to him. In this way you will help to control his shock, which is a very serious part of any accident and can even kill irrespective of other injuries.

The Safety of the Victim

Next, look around you. Are you and the victim in a safe place, or could a further accident happen to either of you? Are you protected from falling rocks from above? If you are directly below a path or a track, any passing walker could easily dislodge a stone. If you hear any rock movement above you, resist the instinct to see what is happening and NEVER LOOK UP. Instead, protect yourself by putting your head in your lap, with your hands over your head, or throw yourself flat against the mountainside head downwards, protecting your head with your hands, so that if you are directly in the path of the rock and cannot escape it, it may bounce over you. Better still, adopt a crouching position behind a rock which would take the force of the blow. If there is a real enough danger of falling rocks and there are boulders lying near by that you can carry, try to build a makeshift wall to protect the victim.

If the ground where the casualty is lying is very steep, there may be a risk of him rolling over an edge or even starting to roll down the hillside. This is especially important if he is unconscious or moving in an uncontrolled jerky fashion, as he might if he were suffering from a fit. If you are on a scree slope where this is a possibility, wedge a rucksack under the casualty to stop him from sliding.

The Importance of Shelter

If the weather is very bad, you will have to consider sheltering the victim. If you are in an exposed place and he is conscious and not too seriously injured, you can help move him to a more sheltered spot. Big boulders and rocky overhangs provide good protection, but make sure that they are safe secure places and not likely to increase the danger you are already in. If the victim is unconscious, he must not be moved, because you may kill him in the process. The only time you should move an unconscious victim is when his life is in very grave danger if he stays where he is. Instead, construct shelter round him.

In winter it is very important that the casualty does not die of exposure in addition to his other injuries, and a vital part of your first aid lies in keeping him warm. If the ground under him is wet or marshy, he will rapidly lose any heat he has into the ground, and you must insulate him as best you can, by putting waterproof material and any spare clothing underneath his body. You must also keep him dry, which is not such a problem if you have with you a large plastic exposure bag in your rucksack. A suitable bag would be 7 feet by 3 feet, of 120-gauge polythene or thicker. You can buy these bags at shops which sell climbing and walking gear. Use all your ingenuity to make whatever form of shelter you can.

If it is summer time, you must still guard against exposure or hypothermia (see pages 134–44) in bad weather because it can, and has, occurred during every month of the year in Britain. The shock following an accident makes a person more susceptible and less resistant to the effects of cold and wet, so although hypothermia is the last thing you would normally think of at the height of summer, don't let the unexpectedness of it overtake you.

In the other extreme, if the weather is very hot and sunny, protect your victim from the direct rays of the sun by making some sort of shade for him. He probably has enough problems already without heatstroke and sunburn.

While you are making the victim as comfortable as you can, think ahead. Wherever you are stranded with him, you will probably be stuck there for the next two hours or so, or even longer if you are in a remote place. What is the weather likely to do in that time? It may not be raining or snowing now, but could it be in three hours' time? Bear this in mind when making any sort of shelter, because, if the wind is blowing directly into your chosen spot, it could be bringing driving rain or snow before long.

These instructions may seem out of place in a first-aid manual, but they are an essential part of mountain first aid and are within the capabilities of anyone. Don't think they are trivial. After all, you could give the most brilliant and complicated first-aid treatment, strapping up broken limbs and dressing wounds, but it would all be pointless if the casualty died in the meantime from something as simple and devastating as the cold. Even if protection from the cold and wet is all that you can do for a victim, it may be the most important thing. For this reason it should be given priority over anything but the most urgent first aid necessary to save life.

Should I Give a Drink?

Very often this is the first request that a conscious casualty makes. At home, the traditional answer to all troubles, physical or mental, is a 'nice cup of tea'. It's warm, familiar and comforting, so, quite naturally, when people become troubled in a strange environment they turn to the simplest best-loved remedies used at home. When help is only a matter of minutes away, the question doesn't usually arise, but with the prospect of a long wait ahead, a cup of tea, coffee, soup or even plain water may be very attractive. Although medical opinion is divided on the benefits of giving drinks in individual cases, on one point their verdict is unanimous:

NEVER, NEVER GIVE AN ALCOHOLIC DRINK OF ANY SORT.

Forget about St Bernard dogs carrying flasks of life-giving brandy round their necks to snow-stranded travellers in the Alps. A nip of spirits given to a person suffering from hypothermia could kill him by causing a sudden rush of warm blood to the cold outer surfaces of the body, which in turn could produce a fatal loss of heat from the vital inner core, which heats and sustains all the essential organs of the body. *Alcohol is of no benefit in any case and can even cause death.*

The question need not concern you at all if you have no Thermos flask and no access to fresh, drinkable water. Nor need you worry about it if the casualty does not ask for a drink. But if he does, you will have to be very attentive, because, while in many cases a drink can be of enormous psychological value and some physical benefit as well, there are particular instances when it can be very harmful and should not be given. Because the problem is rather complicated, the subject of giving a drink is dealt with under the relevant sections for specific injuries and illnesses in Part Three. If you are in any doubt at all, the answer must always be 'No'.

You may wonder what sort of harm a drink could do.

In cases where injuries are very serious, it may be necessary to give the victim a general anaesthetic as soon as he reaches hospital. If a drink has been given not too long before, there is a danger that the patient could choke if he should vomit while under anaesthetic. In some forms of injury, especially to the pelvis and lower regions of the body, it may be very uncomfortable for the victim to pass water, and giving him a drink won't improve this difficulty. Further, giving a drink to anybody seriously injured is not an easy thing to do, and it increases the risk of choking and vomiting. Even if it is permissible to give a drink in a particular case, always make sure that the victim is fully conscious and not likely to pass out.

However, there are occasions when giving a drink is beneficial, for example, in cases of heat exhaustion or cramp. Follow the guidelines given for specific conditions throughout the book. If you have to fetch water from a stream, try to make sure that it is pure by using liquid from swift-flowing streams as far above the nearest known cattle, sheep, camp sites or human dwellings as possible. Water from stagnant lakes or mountain tarns could easily be impure and only add to the victim's problems. When giving tea or coffee, use sugar or glucose in it to help produce energy and warmth and reduce the effects of shock.

The Removal of Clothing

In assessing the victim's injuries, in some cases it may be necessary to remove his clothing. This can present problems in wet or cold conditions. The preservation of body heat is then vital: whenever possible removal of clothing should be avoided. For example, if you suspect that there may be bleeding from an area concealed by clothing, it is better to feel very gently inside the garments, or just open them enough to investigate rather than disturbing the victim by taking the garments off. If you consider the removal of clothing is unavoidable, undress the suspected part of the body as quickly as possible and try not to damage any clothing in the process. Cutting may, however, be necessary in cases where injuries have caused a limb or joint to become distorted and swell, making undressing difficult. Serious fractures, also, can make removal of clothing ex-

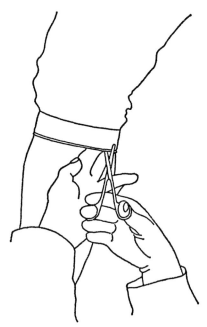

Fig. 5. Removal of clothing by cutting.

tremely painful and perhaps dangerous. In such cases use your sharp scissors to expose the injury rather than increase the victim's discomfort by fumbling with sleeves or trouser legs. Cut in a straight line and fold the garments back. The two pieces of material can be drawn back together again when first aid is complete and held in place by a little sticky tape. This will keep body heat loss to a minimum.

How Serious Are the Injuries?

The condition of the victim is not always immediately apparent. You may actually see a rock crashing down from the scree slope above and striking the victim, or you may see him fall, and in such cases some injuries may be visible or obvious. But other injuries may not, and a life may depend on your ability to discover the full extent of any damage or illness.

In most cases, it takes a doctor to be able to look at an injured or sick person and make an accurate judgement of how bad things are or what complications may follow. As an inexperienced first-aider, you cannot be expected to make this sort of decision, and if you did you might be wrong anyway. But don't give up immediately. You can still try to assess the damage in order to give what help you can; also, in a severe case, you can provide the medical expert with a carefully recorded and timed history of any changes in the condition of the victim which may help him to detect unseen injuries more quickly.

Don't be daunted by your lack of training. Your own eyes, nose, ears and touch will often spot the relevant clues if you have some idea of what to look for. Some of the clues may seem confusing or ambiguous, and you may not know just what they mean. But take a mental note of them all the same, because they may make sense to someone else.

How the investigation is carried out depends on whether the victim is conscious or unconscious.

The Conscious Victim

The conscious casualty is relatively simple to investigate. Nobody can guide you to the source of the trouble more accurately than the victim himself, so ask him. Use the following course of action:

1. Ask the casualty if he is in pain, and where that pain is. The area that he points to is the place to start looking.

If it is necessary to remove clothing, refer to pages 31–2 for the most efficient method.

2. Handle the injured place gently but firmly.

3. Make sure that there are no injuries which may be hidden. Sometimes when a person is in great pain it is difficult for him to locate exactly where it is coming from, and sometimes nerve action can refer the pain away from the seat of the trouble to an undamaged part.

4. Examine the casualty all over his body thoroughly by running your hands gently but firmly over him. Start at the head and neck, work your way down the spine and trunk, and then feel the arms and legs. As you do this, keep in your mind the concept of a body as two matching halves, roughly divided lengthways down the front and back. Keep comparing the two halves, and it will be easier to spot any distortion between the normal uninjured side and the damaged half. This procedure may not be infallible if the casualty has a natural deformity, such as a curvature of the spine, or any physical abnormality resulting from an old injury, or a disease such as polio. To save yourself any confusion, you can check this point with the victim before you go any further.

5. Look at the skin, and feel it. Notice in particular what sort of colour it is. It may be pale and clammy, or it might be very flushed. This might not be of much significance to you, but it may be a vital clue to an expert, who uses even the smallest details as indications of what is happening inside the body. To show how important these fine details are, take the case of serious head injuries. Often a victim who has suffered concussion, or a brain shaking, will look very white and feel cold and clammy. But if a bone is pressing on his brain after the jolt and he is suffering from compression, he may look flushed and feel hot to touch. This may be far too fine a delineation of diagnosis for you, but the information could help a doctor enormously. In the same way, notice how deeply or shallowly the victim is breathing, and, if you can find the pulse (see pages 35, 57), whether it is irregular, strong or weak. To find a wrist pulse,

feel with your fingers on the underside of the wrist on the thumb side about half an inch in. Feel gently, not pressing too hard. To locate the carotid pulse, feel with the finger-tips on the left side of the windpipe below the jawline. It is impossible to generalize on the special significance of

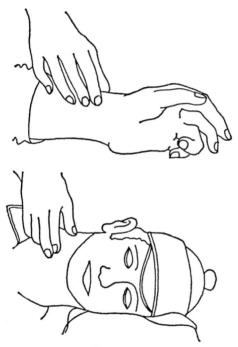

Fig. 6. Finding a pulse.

each of these details, because they may mean quite different things in different cases, so they are dealt with individually when each injury and illness is described. Simply take note of them, and then refer to the condition that you think you might be dealing with and see if the symptoms match the descriptions.

6. Don't get carried away with text-book knowledge and

technicalities so that you forget to listen to what the casualty can tell you. His information is the most important of all.

The Unconscious Victim

If the casualty is unconscious, the task of diagnosis is more difficult, requiring greater observation. This is what you should do:

1. Make sure that the casualty is breathing, and nothing is blocking his air passage. It can happen that an unconscious person dies not of his injuries, such as loss of blood, or shock, but quite simply because he chokes while he is unconscious and not in control of his voluntary actions. This is a tragic and unnecessary way to die, so don't neglect to check this point at the beginning, and thereafter to keep a constant and vigilant watch. If the casualty is choking or not breathing, clear the airway (see page 58) and start assisted breathing if necessary (see pages 59–61).

2. Feel all over the body for abnormalities, comparing each side, as already described in the case of conscious casualties, but let your exploration take in more detail. Feel over and under the victim for any dampness which might mean bleeding or incontinence. The blood may lead you to an injury you cannot see very easily, and if the casualty has passed water this may mean he has severe injuries to his pelvis. If you find areas of bleeding, control them immediately by pressing firmly over the wound with a thick dressing. Refer to page 71 for control of bleeding.

3. You may not know at this stage why the victim is unconscious, but the following observations will help you to judge if he is seriously ill, though they may not provide a diagnosis, since specific abnormalities cannot indicate one simple specific explanation. What you can establish is whether certain regular functions are working abnormally. The more extreme the departure from the normal, the greater the seriousness of the case.

(*a*) Breathing: The average rate in an adult human is about 20 times a minute. Generally a rate of under 15 is dangerously slow, while a rate of over 25 times a minute is far too rapid. If the accident or illness happens during very strenuous activity and you examine the victim immediately after the incident, allow a little time for him to establish a more normal breathing pattern when he has stopped panting after the exertion.

(*b*) Pulse: The average pulse rate is about 80–90 beats a minute in an adult who is not under physical strain. Normally, a rate of 40 beats or under, or 120 or over, per minute is dangerously abnormal.

(*c*) Face and skin: Notice the colour of the cheeks, and if they are particularly pale, or waxy-looking, or bluish in tinge, this may indicate serious injuries or illness. Brightly flushed, rosy cheeks may indicate the same. It helps if you know the victim well enough to have noticed what his normal colouring is, so that any extreme change will show more clearly that he is in danger.

(*d*) Pupils of the eyes: These can tell you quite a lot. In extreme cases, they show whether a victim is already dead. In death, the pupils of the eyes appear very enlarged, and the eyes open very wide and staring. If you can see obvious injuries to the head, a simple test will tell you how bad things are. Close the eyes of the casualty, and cover them with your hand. Then slowly open the eyes and watch the pupils to see if they respond to light, as illustrated in Figure 26 (page 126). A torch can be helpful in checking this response. In normal circumstances, they should get smaller. If they remain enlarged and dilated, this may indicate brain damage. Compare the size of both pupils, one with the other, and remember what you see. If a casualty is this seriously injured, there is very little you can do beyond giving an accurate history when a doctor arrives.

(*e*) Head: Look very gently for any blood in the hair which may indicate a head injury.

(*f*) Eyes, ears, nose and mouth: Look for any signs of blood or injury, but remember that what you see may sometimes be misleading. For example, an inexperienced first-aider might interpret a discharge of blood or fluid from the ear as indicating an injury to the ear itself; to the expert, it could point to a very serious head injury. You cannot always accept symptoms at face value – and they may be more than skin deep.

Keeping a Record

The importance of keeping an accurate record of what is happening to an injured person has already been stressed, but what sort of information should you relate? A written report is more accurate and reliable than memory. So note on paper the time, and describe the condition of the following: breathing, pulse, colour of the skin, warmth of the body, pupils of the eyes. Check these every few minutes, and write down any changes which occur or any new abnormality. If a doctor arrives with a rescue party, hand the paper over directly. If not, make sure that the information does not get lost and that it reaches the right person as soon as possible.

Mystery Illnesses

This book can cover only the commoner types of mountain accident or illness. Were it three times longer, it still could not offer a diagnosis and solution to every conceivable incident you may encounter. This does not mean, however, that there is nothing you can do when you do not know what is wrong.

An unidentifiable crisis may start typically with the victim stopping, clutching his head, chest, stomach or back and refusing to move. Assuming that he has not hurt himself or been stung or bitten, and that he is not diabetic, epileptic or suffering from an allergy, there are endless possibilities. It may be anything from migraine to appendicitis or a perforated ulcer, or simply wind, indigestion, constipation or just a vivid imagination. In other words, it could be trivial or it could be serious. You would probably be able to tell how serious it was only if the victim actually collapsed.

Don't worry if neither you nor the victim can recognize the trouble. Even if you could, you would be unable to treat conditions of this nature on the hills. Don't, however, dismiss the problem and try to force the victim to carry on against his will. What may appear trivial to you may be causing real anxiety to the victim, and this may impair his physical performance which could in itself cause additional problems later. Stop and rest for a while, giving the basic first aid of comfort, reassurance, and warmth and shelter if necessary. If the illness is not serious, the chances are that there will be a return of strength enabling the victim to continue the walk before long, or at least to return to safety.

However, if pain increases or there is no improvement after half an hour's rest, you will have to consider sending for help, or going yourself. In this situation, don't hesitate for fear that you may be causing an unnecessary waste of time and effort. Even if the illness proves to have been trivial after all, you will have acted correctly in making sure that expert help is at hand just in case the problem turned out to be something serious.

Follow the guidelines in Part Two if going for help, and if you are in any doubt about the advisability of giving food or drink to the victim, don't.

Deciding Whether to Send for Help

Apart from mystery illnesses there are other aspects of taking a decision about calling out rescue services. There are those for whom mistaken pride in their own independence and abilities may make them scorn the need for help and, worse still, impose their views on other members of the party. These are the people who 'know these hills like the back of my hand' and who tell hypothermia victims to 'snap out of it' and give them large doses of brandy. At the other extreme, there are those who would rather suffer prolonged agony than be what they consider a nuisance to others. Both attitudes can be extremely dangerous. They should be ignored.

Over-confidence in one's own first-aid ability can also prove disastrous. No matter how much theory has been absorbed and how much practice has been done, the real thing can be horrific enough to render the inexperienced first-aider totally incompetent. There is a great deal of difference between a neat book illustration of clean, expertly dressed and splinted broken arms and legs, and an actual splintered bone poking through raw and gory flesh. Don't be ashamed because you need help to do what you thought you could do yourself.

Remember that in cases where a victim is completely immobilized by severe injuries or illness, makeshift and inexpert carrying can seriously affect the chances of survival and certainly increase suffering and shock. When there are serious injuries which don't in themselves prevent the victim from walking, bear in mind that the pain and loss of agility which they will almost certainly cause will impair the victim's chances of continuing to walk without further mishap, however good the first aid.

Such cases, and also cases of hypothermia, heart attack, loss of blood, head, chest and spinal injuries must be *carried* off the hill. This job should not be undertaken without proper equipment and trained personnel in adequate numbers. Rescue teams consider that eight fit men are needed to carry one victim over any distance to safety.

In less serious cases, a victim may tell you that he prefers to walk down unaided. He will probably be the best judge of his ability to do so, and unless there are other factors such as bad weather conditions, or very rough ground, to consider, you should let him continue, accompanied preferably by at least two people. Then, if he gets into difficulty, one can go for help and the other give first aid.

Within every recognized walking and climbing area of Britain, teams of trained and experienced local rescuers exist. Some are drawn from the services or the police, but many of them are unpaid volunteers who join rescue organizations out of enthusiasm for hill pursuits. They share the same interests as the victims they help and they understand how easy it is for problems to arise. They take a pride in providing a fast, efficient and sympathetic skilled service. For them a rescue call-out is not a nuisance; it is a new challenge to be met. You should never hesitate on grounds of causing trouble to call on their help. In addition to their own training in first aid to an advanced level, they possess all the equipment necessary to carry out a well-organized and speedy rescue, including survival apparatus, special stretchers and often radio. They can summon a doctor quickly if needed, and they can also alert the R.A.F. Search and Rescue Helicopter Service for emergency evacuation of a victim if necessary. In short, their capabilities and technical equipment will be far superior to anything you can do for the casualty, once they have arrived on the scene of the incident.

All this organization and help will cost you nothing more than the donation you may like to give the rescue team funds when the job is over. So if you cannot perform the necessary first aid, or if the victim obviously needs carrying, or if it is too painful for him to try to walk, or if the weather and general conditions would make it dangerous for him to do so, call the rescue team.

Emergency Action Quick Reference

1. Whoever goes for help must know:

(*a*) Precise location of incident (e.g. map reference, name of crag, name and pitch number of climbing route, fell side, gully, landmarks).

(*b*) Time of incident.

(*c*) Nature of injuries.

(*d*) Whether victim needs personal medications (e.g., insulin). This information should be WRITTEN DOWN rather than memorized.

2. Send more than one person if possible.

3. In a party of only two, an unconscious victim must not be left alone unless absolutely necessary (see page 45).

4. The bearer of the message for help should head for the most quickly accessible inhabited location and CONTACT THE POLICE. Once there, he should not return to the accident scene unless or until instructed, and should follow any instructions given by the police or rescue team.

The size of groups has a bearing on mountain safety. Obviously, the larger the group, the greater the chances of someone meeting with an accident. Ideally, the size of a walking party should range from three to about ten people.

A minimum of three means that if one person suffers an accident and cannot get down the hill without assistance, then there are two others to deal with the problem – one to go for help and the other to stay with the victim and give first aid. With only two, the situation becomes more difficult, and for the solo walker it is harder still. Conversely, parties of over ten with only one leader are liable to suffer as a result of other factors. It is not an uncommon sight to observe groups of thirty or even more walking the hills. Those thirty are individuals with varying ages, interests, abilities, strength, fitness, stamina and speed, and such a large group will tend to separate, with an advance party striding on ahead and the stragglers, sometimes miles behind, trying to keep up. Less experienced leaders don't always see the potential risk in allowing a group to disintegrate. In this way people get anxious, and even lost. This warning is especially relevant when conditions are bad. In time, everybody can be affected to a greater or lesser degree, and hypothermia, which comes on suddenly, could cause, and has on occasion caused, total collapse among many group members in quick succession. The more people in trouble, the bigger the problems of rescue. So try to confine groups to manageable numbers, particularly in the case of parties of children when the ratio of leaders to children should be roughly one to five.

Parties of Three or More

If an accident happens to somebody in a sensibly sized party of between three and ten, the procedure for going for help is fairly simple as long as you remember certain common-sense rules. Decide first who will go, bearing in mind fitness, tiredness and knowledge of the area.

Next, write down all the relevant details of the incident. You should include the precise location of the accident (using a six-figure map reference, and noting any sizable landmarks and compass bearings, if possible) and the name of the rock face, climb or hillside you may be on; how many people are injured and with what type of injuries; and whether the victim is a special case requiring personal medications such as insulin.

Note the time of the accident, and indicate the spot where the victim lies with a marker of any coloured material you have. The bright orange 'Dayglo' anoraks are ideal. It is always as well to have some brightly coloured item with you on the hills for this purpose. If it can be done without wasting time and if suitable material is available, whoever is sent for help should leave a trail of markers so that rescuers can follow them to the accident scene; but these are not much use unless they stand out against the natural background. If it is snowing, or likely to snow, the markers should be left so that they will stick up out of the snow. If the party is large enough, send two or three people to get help – this will lessen the risk of anything happening to a single messenger which might prevent his reaching help. If necessary enlist the help of anyone you meet. Your objective is to reach a telephone, where you should dial 999 and ask for the police. Tell them what is written on your piece of paper, with details of where the accident has happened and also where you are ringing from. While you are waiting for the police to call out the nearest mountain rescue team, don't start back up the hill unless you have been told to. Stay exactly where you have arranged to meet the rescuers and resist the temptation to rush back to the victim. You could get lost on the way, and the team may not be able to locate the victim without your guidance.

Parties of Two

If you have accepted the risks involved in walking with only one other person, the decisions in the event of an accident become more difficult. Action will depend on whether the victim is conscious or unconscious.

If your companion is *unconscious*, then it is very dangerous to leave him or her alone, and in most cases the best possible action is to remain with the casualty and hope to attract the attention of someone. If you have a whistle or torch, use the international distress signal with both or either. This is six long blasts or flashes in quick succession, repeated once a minute and continued until rescuers arrive. Be as accurate as you can, so that people below will not confuse your cry for help with other lights and sounds on the hill. Each year rescue teams deal with dozens of false alarms involving car headlights, fireworks, bright stars, aircraft lights and even falling meteors. With all these attracting attention, your torch light may be explained away by anybody who happens to notice it unless you are exact and persistent. Shout as loudly as you can if you think anyone might hear you. This, incidentally, is the reason why one should never shout unnecessarily on the hills. People may think you are in trouble when you are not, and may risk their lives trying to help you.

In a very remote area, where you can assume that your isolation is almost total, it is clearly impossible to remain and hope to attract attention. You both may die of hypothermia if you sit waiting for help long enough. You can only judge this for yourself at the time, but if you think it very unlikely that anyone will see or hear you within a couple of hours, you will have to leave the unconscious victim. In such a case, carefully move the person into a sheltered spot; or, if he is very badly injured, build a shelter round him. If he is lying on a steep slope or ledge, use whatever is available to prevent him from falling. It may be possible to use a rucksack or rope to attach him to something solid like a rock. Leave a note explaining what has happened and what you are doing, and then proceed down the hill, leaving markers, and dial 999 when you reach the nearest telephone.

If the victim is *conscious* the best thing to do is leave him and go for help after giving first aid and making him as comfortable as you can. Give him all the spare clothing and food that you have, as well as your whistle, and also your torch if you can find your way without it. Make sure that he understands that he must not attempt to start down the hill on his own, and mark the place clearly before you go. If you are alone with a victim in a remote spot, it is pointless, even harmful, to try to drag or half carry the person to safety down the hill. You may kill him in the process and exhaust yourself as well. Injured bodies are heavy to carry over rough ground. Mountain rescue teams allow at least eight strong men to rescue one victim, carrying the stretcher in turns.

Walking or Climbing Alone

Clearly, a solo walker or climber who suffers a serious accident is unable to send for help. The best chance lies in trying to attract attention by the methods already described (page 46). This is possible only if injuries have not rendered him unconscious. If he is unconscious, obviously there is no way he can get attention, and unless you are strongly motivated to accept the considerable risks in solo mountaineering, the best advice is never to go alone. If you do, at least ensure before departure that someone knows your route and expected time of return.

Rescue Posts and Stretcher Boxes

For many years before rescue teams came into being, the only available first-aid help in many hill areas was situated at rescue posts and stretcher boxes. The rescue posts are still administered by the Mountain Rescue Committee, a body of representatives from mountaineering clubs and other groups associated with hill pursuits. They are supervised by local people, including hostel wardens and hoteliers, and their locations are shown on some maps. Each post, usually housed in a shed, contains such basic equipment as a stretcher, bandages, splints, a stove, lanterns, Thermos flasks, exposure bags and blankets. Stretcher boxes are placed in strategic spots on the hills, often near a summit, and they contain limited equipment. Anybody can open the box and help himself to the contents.

These unmanned posts and boxes have been life-savers in the past before permanent rescue teams were formed, but nowadays their existence causes concern in some quarters because inexpert rescuers are tempted to organize their own rescue operations even though trained and experienced rescue teams can do a much safer job. The main danger arises in cases of serious injury. If expert first-aid knowledge is not available, potentially fatal conditions such as chest,

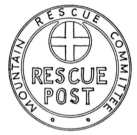

Fig. 7. Rescue post sign.

spinal and head injuries may not be discovered before the victim is placed on a stretcher by his friends and man-handled clumsily down the hill. Many such cases should not be moved at all until proper medical treatment can be given on the spot, and even rescue teams may prefer to have evacuation carried out by helicopter if possible to save vital time.

On the other hand, if a victim is immobilized by a shin or ankle injury and has suffered no other damage, it should be within the capabilities of a reasonable number of his companions to bring him down on a stretcher from a rescue post if one is available near by, thus saving a great deal of time and effort on the part of the rescue team.

A careful assessment therefore must be made of the full extent of any injuries, taking into account such factors as shock, before deciding not to bother the rescue team and 'do it yourself'. In case of doubt, the best course is to call the team. It would be irresponsible to deny a victim access to the best available resources when his life or future health may depend on it. The only exception to this rule would be in those cases where leaving the victim where he is might lead to his death from hypothermia. If a decision is taken to move a victim by means of a stretcher from a box or post, it is a wise precaution to send for help at the same time, so that, if difficulties or complications arise, a rescue team will be able to assist by meeting you half way.

Rescue posts and stretcher boxes sometimes contain morphine ampoules for the relief of severe pain, though this drug is often removed, together with other items, by vandals. If morphine is available, it must NEVER be used if there are head, chest or spinal injuries because it may interfere with breathing. It must also never be used on an unconscious victim.

Part Three   FIRST-AID PRACTICE

So far, we have dealt with general care of accident victims and common-sense sequences of action. The rest of the book deals with the treatment of particular incidents and injuries. Some of these have been recorded by rescue teams only once or twice in the last few years, and they may seem rather obscure and improbable. But every condition described has occurred in Britain on the hills some time within living memory, some of them frequently. They may be familiar to rescuers, but for the inexperienced first-aider they can be very alarming. So bear in mind the following principles before reading in detail what to do about individual cases.

In most circumstances, you will have to make your own judgement as well as using the information in this book. If you are not sure about what to do, do nothing at all, unless there is danger of immediate death. Doing nothing can be as important a part of first aid as actually doing something, because if you do the wrong thing it might turn out to be far more damaging than if you had left well alone.

Some of the procedures described may be too complicated for you. Know your limitations. For example, a commonly used method of making a fracture casualty more comfortable is to immobilize the broken limb by strapping it to uninjured parts of the body. For a broken leg the conventional first aid would be to pad the hollow between the two legs and strap the bad one to the good one to stop it from moving and causing pain. If you feel competent to do this, and you really are making the victim more comfortable, go ahead in the way described. But if you feel at all uneasy about treating a person in considerable pain in this way, especially when he indicates that he would really rather not be touched at all, it may be much better first aid to do nothing except keep him warm and comforted. Obviously, with an injury like that he is unable to walk down, and you will presumably both be waiting for a stretcher party to arrive. That rescue party will be trained in first aid, and will have immobilized fractures by the dozens over the years. The casualty won't lose much by waiting for somebody to come and do the job competently. The whole point of immobilization is to make being carried down the hill more comfortable. It is often not needed until the stretcher arrives.

Never use the directions and advice in any first-aid manual as laws to be followed at all costs. First aid is about helping people; those people are all individual beings in different kinds of trouble, and no two emergencies are ever quite the same. What may be suitable for one case might be inappropriate for another.

Be guided by the victim himself if he is conscious. Whatever the book tells you to do in particular cases may be correct in theory, but in practice it is worth only as much as the comfort and general good it does for the casualty.

If the advice in the book seems to be going contrary to a casualty's own natural inclinations, you must stop, think and decide for yourself whether you are doing more harm than good. It has been known for keen first-aiders, armed with their books and graphic illustrations on how to treat fractures, or what position a certain injury should be kept in, to descend on the poor victim and succeed only in moving him from a position in which he was quite content to the 'correct' one in which he was extremely uncomfortable.

Whatever the book says, if somebody prefers to stay as he is and if his life is not in any danger by leaving him, let him lie as he is. His comfort is far more important than trying to make him look like a drawing in a first-aid book.

Because the approach of this book is intentionally un-complicated, do not make the mistake of thinking that first aid is easy. It is not. Sometimes it is physically exhausting; often it is very unpleasant, and not for the squeamish. Most of us, however tough we imagine we are, have a shocked reaction when we face a gory sight or a person in great pain. But even if you have never encountered any such emergency before, be confident in the knowledge that, in the event, most people manage to overcome their own repugnance and fear, and rise to the occasion. Many of us do not know our own reserves of strength until we actually have to use them.

Incidents on the hills requiring help and first aid are not restricted to accidents only. A sudden illness can occur just as easily on a mountain as it can at home. In fact, the physical strain involved in climbing or walking, combined perhaps with the stress of anxiety, can precipitate an illness which might not otherwise occur. For instance, heart attacks happen with depressing frequency, unaccustomed exertion acting as a trigger to an attack which may have been going to occur sooner or later anyway. The anxieties that inexperienced hill walkers can feel if the weather is bad or the mist comes down, or if they are unable to keep pace with others in a party, could contribute to just such an unexpected emergency. Remember also that the physical challenge of the mountains may reduce your natural capacity to cope with the crisis or withstand the illness, so mountain first aid must include knowledge of how to deal with these kinds of emergency.

Apart from anxieties, other quite unforeseeable emer-gencies have hit people on the hills. Whatever elaborate preparations you make for your adventure, you cannot fore-see the sandwich with the wasp in it waiting to be swallowed or the bee which decides to sting the only person in the group who is allergic to bee stings. The more foolhardy in the party may decide to sample the local fungi, or drink from a stream only yards below the spot picked by a now dead and decaying animal to have his last drink . . . and the consequences could be sudden and dramatic. So if you are inclined to think that some of the illnesses mentioned are highly unlikely or plain impossible, remember – they have actually happened. Be ready to cope with the more bizarre incidents. After all, the very nature of an accident is its unpredictability and unexpectedness.

For ease of reference, the incidents in this chapter are dealt with in alphabetical order rather than in terms of urgency, importance or frequency with which they occur. In case of emergency it is, we repeat, far better to have read the book and know the general idea of the procedure than to have to look everything up on the spot. However, in the case of an accident or illness which may prove fatal, a quick reference for emergency action is provided.

ARTIFICIAL RESUSCITATION

If you do not know the techniques of artificial resuscitation before you need to use them, you may well be too late. It is considered worthwhile to give below a quick emergency reference, but this will be of little use unless you already know the detailed procedure in the text which follows.

Emergency Action Quick Reference

IF BREATHING HAS STOPPED, check also for HEART STOP.
IF HEART IS STILL BEATING, CLEAR AIR-WAY. If breathing does not start, begin MOUTH-TO-MOUTH ASSISTED BREATHING.
IF HEART HAS ALSO STOPPED begin CARDIAC COMPRESSION. CLEAR AIRWAY if obstructed and combine CARDIAC COMPRESSION with MOUTH-TO-MOUTH ASSISTED BREATHING.

To check whether BREATHING has stopped:

  1. Listen at mouth or nose, and/or
  2. Hold shiny article such as tin lid or compass glass to mouth and look for misting.

To check whether HEART has stopped:

  1. Feel for pulse in carotid (neck) artery, and/or
  2. Unfasten thick outer garments and listen with ear to chest.

To clear AIRWAY:

  1. Lay victim on his side, with head lower than body, to drain airway.
  2. Remove any obstruction or fluid in mouth with hooked finger.
  3. If tongue is causing obstruction, clear by tilting head and holding jaw forwards.
  4. If now no apparent obstruction, but breathing does not start, strike sharply between shoulder blades, then recheck for any obstructing object and remove.
  5. If still no breathing, begin assisted breathing.

General

Artificial resuscitation is not only the most difficult first-aid technique but also the most important. A life may depend on your quick action. The one question you need not ask yourself, as you have to in most other first aid, is whether inexperienced attempts will do more harm than good. Once a person stops breathing or his heart stops beating, he cannot be any worse off, whatever damage may inadvertently be caused in your efforts to revive him. During the four minutes after a victim stops breathing or his heart stops beating, there is a chance to save his life; after that time the chances are slim, but it is always worth trying. So, to be effective at all, your life-saving actions must start as quickly as possible, and you will have to get it right first time. There will be no time to stop and think about whether you are doing the right thing correctly.

There are two methods of resuscitation, and it may be necessary to use both at once. The first involves breathing artificially for the victim by blowing air into his chest to encourage him to start breathing again for himself. The second method involves regular compression of the heart if it is no longer beating, and is usually known as external cardiac compression or massage. This action stimulates the heart in an attempt to make it start functioning again on its own. The technique is extremely tiring and not always effective; if the heart is not beating anyway, the victim is in such a bad way that his chances of recovery are slight. Many first-aid experts would be anxious at the prospect of the untrained first-aider carrying out cardiac compression on a victim with the help of only written instructions, and there is some controversy over the encouragement of the use of this method by the inexperienced. Some experts say that it should never be attempted by someone who hasn't practised it in a first-aid class. If it is done incorrectly, it can cause quite serious internal injuries. As the alternative is almost certain death, others think that any possible damage is an acceptable risk. We consider the last opinion is correct in the isolation of the hills. When a person collapses in a street only minutes away from an ambulance and trained first-aiders, there may be a case for hesitating for a few seconds to find out if anybody near by knows how to do it better than you. But on the hills there won't be a passing off-duty doctor, nurse or ambulanceman, so the victim's life will rest on your decision whether to have a go or not.

When Might It Be Needed?

The most common types of accident which may cause stoppage of heart or breathing include: a fall or blow on the head; crushing or suffocation by rocks, snow or ice; choking or strangulation by rope, clothing or rucksack while climbing; insufficient ventilation in tents while cooking; heart attacks, fits and severe shock following loss of blood.

Suspect stoppage of breathing or heart following any of the above incidents.

How to Tell if Breathing Has Stopped

You can tell quite easily if someone is having difficulty breathing. He will struggle to get air in and out of his lungs, and the muscles in his neck will bulge with the effort, but there will be little rise and fall of his chest. Or his breathing, such as it is, may be noisy, or very slow, or have a bubbling sound. Gradually he will go a greyish-blue colour round his lips, ears and fingernails. If you suspect that he has stopped breathing altogether either listen by putting your ear next to his nose or mouth to see if you can feel or hear any air movement; or, if you have a mirror or tin lid to hand, place it over the victim's mouth for a second and if he is breathing the condensation will show on the shiny surface. At the same time feel underneath his clothing just under his chest to see if there is any movement.

How to Tell if the Heart Has Stopped

External warnings of heart stoppage are unconsciousness, and a greyish-blue tinge around the lips, ear lobes, tongue and fingernails. Oxygen starvation of the brain will cause enlargement of the pupils of the eyes.

Checking for a Pulse

The wrist pulse, which is the well-known test, may be very weak, and there is a danger that you may feel your own finger pulse at this point and confuse it with the victim's. A better check will be provided by feeling for the carotid pulse by pressing gently on the left side of the windpipe in the neck (see page 35). To be as certain as possible that the heart has stopped, you can also listen with your ear against the victim's chest, having first unfastened any thick outer clothing. If you are certain that there is no heart beat, cardiac compression is necessary.

Resuscitation Procedure

If breathing has stopped or is partially blocked, the airway must first be checked and quickly cleared of any obstruction. This may well restart breathing without the need for further action. The usual causes of obstruction are the back of the tongue, which in an unconscious person may fall back across the airway, or a collection in the airway of vomit, saliva or blood. In addition to these, 'foreign' objects, such as dentures, may have become lodged in the airway after a severe shaking.

To Clear the Airway

1. Turn the casualty on one side with his head lying lower than the rest of his body. This should make the

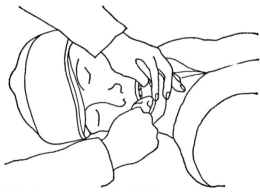

Fig. 8. Clearing the mouth of debris.

tongue fall forward and let any fluid drain by gravity. Then remove any solid obstruction such as dentures and hook out anything else such as vomit and any other fluid. Breathing may then have restarted.

2. If it has not, the falling back of the tongue may still be causing a blockage. Lay the victim on his back. (This is not essential but will make what follows easier.) Place one

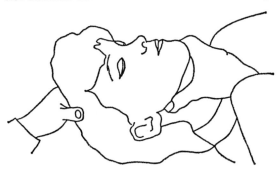

Fig. 9. Jaw-holding.

hand at the back of the casualty's neck and tilt his head back by raising that hand. This will ensure that the windpipe is straight. Then, using both hands, grip each side of the lower jaw, with the little fingers curled behind the angle of the jaw just below each ear. Pull firmly but without jerking to bring the lower jaw forward. This will pull the back of the tongue clear of the airway. This action may well enable breathing to restart.

3. If it does not, mouth-to-mouth assisted breathing must be tried.

Mouth-to-Mouth Assisted Breathing

This can be a distasteful operation, and it may be necessary to overcome your repugnance at contact with the victim's mouth, which could be dirty with blood or vomit. It may help to place a handkerchief or thin gauze dressing between your mouth and the victim's. Then do as follows:

1. Kneel at right angles to the line of the casualty's body at chest level so that you can place your mouth over his. The victim should be lying on his back. Tilt the head back.

2. Pinch his nose closed to prevent air escaping through it.

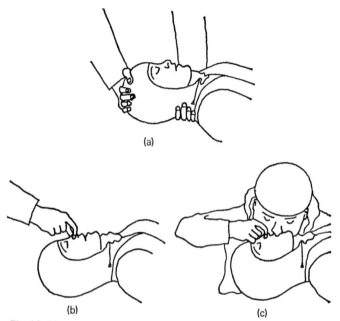

Fig. 10. Mouth-to-mouth assisted breathing : (a) Tilt head back ;
(b) Pinch nose closed ; (c) Form airtight seal and blow.

3. Take a deep breath.

4. Put your open mouth tightly over the casualty's mouth to form an airtight seal. If forming a seal is difficult because of facial injury, you should try applying your mouth to the nose.

5. Blow air into him until you see his chest rise.

6. Take your mouth away so that the lungs can expel the air. This will happen automatically.

7. Repeat actions 5 and 6 once every five seconds.

8. If breathing does not start, check again for airway blockage. If you think there may be something you cannot see causing a blockage, quickly roll the casualty on his side and hit him fairly sharply between the shoulder blades. This may dislodge anything stuck in the throat. Check the mouth again to remove anything dislodged, and begin mouth-to-mouth breathing again.

9. If at any time you notice the stomach starting to bulge as you blow air into the lungs, this means that you are forcing too much air too hard into the lungs and it is escaping into the stomach. This increases the likelihood that the victim will vomit, so press your hand on his stomach to push the air out and be prepared for him to be sick. Push his head gently to one side and be ready to clear his airway out once again with a hooked finger in case of blockage by vomit, before proceeding again with the respiration.

Once breathing has started, roll the casualty onto his side and arrange for his head to be lower than the rest of his body. This is the best position for him to be in to get rid of any secretions which have lodged in his lungs, or to vomit

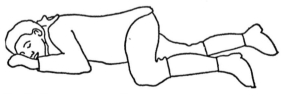

Fig. 11. The recovery position.

without choking. Lay him on his left side with his leg lying straight and draw his other leg up so it is bent at the knee. Make sure his head is resting on one side to prevent choking.

If after a minute of mouth-to-mouth resuscitation breathing does not start, check that the heart is still beating, in the way already described. If it is not, you will have to start cardiac compression as well.

Cardiac Compression (External Heart Massage)

This consists of two stages:

1. The striking stage.
2. The pushing stage.

The Striking Stage

(*a*) Make sure that the victim is lying on his back on firm ground, then strike his chest smartly to the left of the lower part of the breast bone. This may be enough to restart the heart beating. Check to see if there is a heart beat as already described.

(*b*) If there is no heart beat, repeat the striking action every two to three seconds about six times. Then check once again for a heart beat.

(*c*) If nothing has happened, kneel down by the victim and again find the lower half of his breast bone, in preparation for starting the pushing stage of the massage.

The Pushing Stage

(*d*) Put the heel of one hand on this part of the bone, keeping your palm and fingers raised above the chest.

(*e*) Cover this hand with the heel of the other hand, and, with your arms straight, rock forwards, pressing downwards on the bone. For an adult, do this every second, but for a child use a quicker, lighter stroke with one hand only, about 80–90 times a minute.

(*f*) While performing external compression, you must not stop assisted breathing. If you are on your own with the victim, press the breast bone fifteen times, then breathe twice through the victim's mouth to inflate his lungs. If there are two people, let one person do the compression while the other does the mouth-to-mouth assisted breathing and allow five heart compressions and then one deep lung inflation.

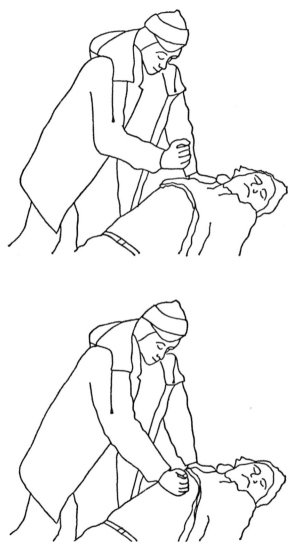

Fig. 12. Cardiac compression : the striking stage.

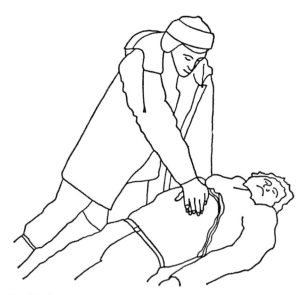

Fig. 13. Cardiac compression: the pushing stage.

Signs of Improvement

Look for the following points:

1. The pupils of the eyes: if the victim is recovering, these should start to respond to light and become less dilated and staring.

2. The carotid (neck) pulse: this will indicate whether the heart beat has been restarted.

3. Skin colour: once the heart starts to pump oxygen back into the bloodstream, the victim should begin to look a more normal, pink colour instead of the bluish-grey tinge noticeable in his face before.

If these signs of improvement are present, it means that

by pressing the chest and breathing into the lungs, you are providing a blood circulation, but you may not have started the heart beating on its own. The only way to tell if you have succeeded in restarting the heart and breathing independently of your artificial resuscitation is to stop and see what happens. Check the pulse and observe breathing. If the pulse is beating but the breathing is not taking place, the assisted breathing will have to be continued. If neither is present, both will have to be artificially restarted.

Signs That the Victim Has Died

1. There will be no change in the size of the dilated eye pupils, the bluish-grey colour of the skin, and there will be no pulse.
2. If you continue resuscitation, you will notice the muscles becoming hard and rigid. This means that rigor mortis has set in after death, and further attempts at resuscitation are futile.

If the victim dies, naturally you will be most upset and distressed, but do not reproach yourself in any way. Even if you carry out the life-saving techniques exactly as directed, this help is extremely limited without more sophisticated equipment, though it is the best that you can do for the victim on the hills.

However, if he recovers, don't let the euphoria you feel at your success cause you to forget the possibility of a further stoppage and collapse. You have achieved only the beginning of your first-aid treatment and not its completion. You must be ready at all times to cope with a sudden relapse. To make sure that this does not happen without your noticing it, keep a regular check on the pulse, pupils of the eyes, skin colour and breathing, and if there is any deterioration in any of these points, you may have to resume resuscitation if heart or breathing stop again.

Reviving a dying person is a complicated matter, as the last few pages will have indicated. If you are ever faced with such a grave crisis, remember that whatever you do should be carried out calmly, steadily and evenly without jerkiness or excessive force. You must find the right pace so that your actions are entirely regular and as similar as possible to the normal, regular actions of the heart and lungs; and, by working smoothly at an even pace, the physical effort involved in mouth-to-mouth assisted breathing and cardiac compression will be less exhausting for you.

ASTHMA

What Is It?

Asthma is a difficulty in breathing caused by a spasm affecting muscles which control air tubes in the lungs. It can be caused either by physical or mental irritants or stress, and attacks can last just a few minutes or as long as twenty-four hours. While not a killer in itself, asthma can cause heart failure.

What Should I Notice?

When someone is having an attack of asthma, he has difficulty in breathing out, and in his efforts to do so he often wheezes or makes a whistling sound. Sufferers become extremely distressed and anxious. An asthmatic person often experiences an attack after he has felt stress or anxiety, for example after a very difficult climb or a steep scramble.

What Can I Do?

The best thing the first-aider can do is to help the victim to help himself. Most asthmatics carry supplies of drugs and inhalants to control the spasm, so feel in the victim's pockets and look in his rucksack for any remedy he may have brought to help himself, and then help him to use it.

Although the attack is most unpleasant and upsetting for the victim, it is rarely dangerous, and it can be minimized if you remember that tension of some sort may have caused it. Remove whatever worry may have set it off. Reassure the victim. Be calm, confident and unexcited.

There is some practical advice, based on the experiences of asthmatics who have actually suffered attacks while walking or climbing, that you can give the victim during an attack. Tell the victim to try to breathe out more fully on each exhalation. Most asthmatics, during an attack, tend to 'pile up' breath, over-inhaling in their desperation to breathe. If you mention this, it may help the victim to be less anxious.

Should I Send for Help?

You cannot decide this until you see how serious the attack is. Sometimes, it may be over very quickly, and the victim will suffer no ill effects if he feels like continuing the day's exercise; or he might prefer to walk slowly down in his own time, with another member of the party. But if the attack is severe or the victim is not carrying an inhalant or drug to control it, send for help immediately.

Can I Give a Drink?

Yes. Give him anything he feels he would like, and do everything you can to restore his confidence and security.

If you are an asthmatic yourself, and feel that you might be prone to an attack on the hills, it would help the leader of your party if you mentioned this to him or her before you start. But if, as leader of a party, you are told of the presence of an asthmatic, don't worry. It is possible to be an extremely powerful athlete and asthmatic as well. Don't try to discourage an asthmatic from enjoying the hills; that is his own decision. Instead, make sure he is carrying the necessary drugs or inhalant in an accessible place.

BITES

SEE INSECT BITES, page 144, and SNAKE BITES, page 157.

BLEEDING

Emergency Action Quick Reference (Heavy Bleeding)

1. Lay victim down on the ground and make a padded dressing with which to apply pressure.
2. Hold pad directly and firmly over the wound.
3. Release pressure every five minutes to check if bleeding has stopped. If not, reapply pad more firmly.
4. If there is no sign of underlying fracture, raise the affected limb and keep it in this position.
5. Treat victim for shock (see page 153).
6. Check that no other areas of external bleeding lie hidden under clothing.

General

Bleeding is a leakage from any of the blood vessels – veins, arteries and capillaries – and is caused when something happens to damage the blood vessel. If you cut your hand on broken glass, you can see blood leaking from your body through the severed vessels. Bleeding of this kind, external bleeding, is simple to recognize. The damage and leakage in blood vessels caused by typical mountain falls is often under the skin or deep inside the body. Internal bleeding is serious, but you cannot see the bleeding, and there may be no sign at all of internal loss of blood.

What is so important about loss of blood? You may think that, with eight pints each, we can afford to lose quite an amount before we are really at risk. But each drop of blood in our bodies is carrying vital supplies of oxygen, glucose and other materials essential to life, and the body very soon starts to feel the ill effects. A healthy adult would probably survive the loss of about 15 per cent of his total blood supply, which works out at about 1·2 pints, but that doesn't take into account either the damage which is causing the bleeding or the drop in blood pressure called shock, which bleeding also causes. Bleeding of any nature is a potentially dangerous threat to life, but fortunately very simple first aid can control it and prevent death by excessive loss of blood.

What Should I Look For?

The most obvious outward signs are easy to see and trace, but when the bleeding is taking place inside the body out of sight, there is very little you can notice. After any serious accident, it is fairly safe to assume that there may be invisible internal bleeding. You cannot actually stop or control it, but you can minimize its effects by treating the victim for shock (see page 153), which is the body's automatic drop in blood pressure when it discovers there is insufficient fluid to pump round.

Deep cuts and gashes are an obvious cause of bleeding, but not the only cases in which bleeding must be treated as a major consideration. Internal bleeding can be caused by a fall or a blow which leaves the outer skin untouched while the blood vessels underneath have been broken and damaged. Bleeding can also be a major factor in fractures, and as a first-aider you may have to control the bleeding from a broken limb before you even consider what to do about the break itself. This is particularly significant in certain types of fracture, especially the femur or thigh bone, because as much blood can escape from the site of this fracture as can pour out of a cut throat after an efficient attempt at suicide. So, whatever the injury, the first problem may be controlling blood loss.

How Can I Tell How Serious the Loss Is?

The simplest way to tell how serious is the loss of blood is to look for obvious signs of shock, even if you cannot see a pool of blood. Serious bleeding causes a sudden drop in blood pressure, and the victim will look very pale as his blood vessels struggle to compensate for the loss and retain what blood is left for the most important internal organs. He may feel cold and clammy, and shiver uncontrollably. If he displays all these signs and there is still no obvious sign of loss, make a thorough check before you decide it is an internal loss that you can do nothing about. You may not have noticed external bleeding, especially if the victim is wearing dark clothing, or if he is obscuring the source of the bleeding by the way in which he is lying on the ground. Use your hands to feel very gently all over him, inside his outer layers of clothing, and, if you feel a damp patch anywhere, examine the area to see what it is. If you don't make this quick inspection, you may miss the chance to save his life by failing to spot the hidden injury.

Another way that you can identify instances of serious bleeding is by the colour of the fluid and the way that it is being pumped out of the damaged vessel. If an artery is cut, it is a break in the tube carrying blood away from the heart. That blood will appear bright scarlet and will escape from the wound in spurts, in the rhythm that the heart is still pumping it. Arteries are very tough, strong tubes and more protected than veins, which carry blood to the heart and are more often the victims of damage than arteries. When a vein is severed, the blood is a much darker colour, and it flows out of the wound more smoothly. In either of these cases, you may have to control the blood loss very quickly to prevent the death of the casualty.

The Tourniquet

The control of bleeding is one of the most controversial issues in first aid, and the argument is centred round the use of the tourniquet. This is a restricting band made of any sort of material which is tied tightly around the limb above the area of bleeding, to prevent blood from reaching that part of the limb at all, and thus preventing any further loss. It used to be standard first-aid practice to train students in the use of tourniquets, but they are now considered to cause such serious side-effects that the harm they can do is thought to outweigh the benefits, and their use has now largely been abandoned. The tourniquet is dangerous because, if it is left on for even as little as half an hour without release, the absence of blood in the limb may destroy it and the bleeding will be controlled, for example, at the high cost of an amputated arm or leg. Tourniquets are really unnecessary and certainly not worth the risk of causing further damage because bleeding can be controlled quite easily by direct pressure without them. On balance, we consider that the dangers inherent in using a tourniquet are far greater than the good they may do, and no reference will be made to them when discussing the methods of controlling bleeding.

How to Control Serious and Minor Bleeding

The same action is appropriate for both:

1. Lay the victim flat on the ground. This helps to reduce blood flow and loss because the heart-beat is slower.

2. Find a sterile dressing in your first-aid kit and use any kind of material to hand, for example triangular bandages, or even a spare sanitary towel, to make a padding behind the dressing.

3. Place the dressing over the wound, and press the padding firmly on top of it directly over the area of bleeding. Release the pressure every five minutes or so to see if the bleeding is being controlled. If it is not, reapply the dressing and padding with more pressure.

4. If you are quite certain that there is no underlying fracture near the wound, gently lift the affected limb in the air as high as the level of the heart. If it is a vein which is

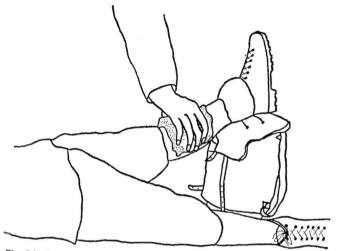

Fig. 14. Control of bleeding by direct pressure and elevation of limb.

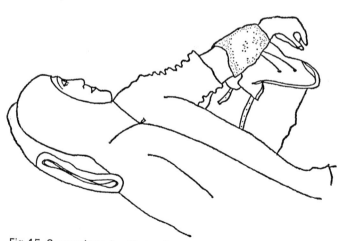

Fig. 15. Supporting raised limb using rucksack.

bleeding, the pressure in the vessel will drop, and the bleeding will stop. Support the raised limb using a rucksack.

5. Once you can see that the bleeding has stopped, the body has then successfully put into operation its own emergency system for stopping further loss. The blood vessels narrow, so that less blood can escape, and the blood itself has its own clotting mechanism which seals the area of the wound and stops the leakage. Once this process has started, be careful not to upset it, or bleeding will start again as before. Let the blood form a clot, and do not dab at it with a bandage or handkerchief in case you dislodge it.

6. Even after the wound has stopped bleeding, make a regular check to ensure that it has not started again.

This technique is not only extremely simple but also highly effective, and as soon as the control is achieved, turn your attention to counteracting the effects of shock.

Can I Give a Drink?

Although a drink may help to reduce shock, generally it is better not to give victims of serious bleeding more than just a sip or two. Serious internal injuries may require surgical repair as soon as possible, in which case nothing should have been taken by mouth for some hours before an anaesthetic is given because of the danger of choking or vomiting while unconscious. However, if you know that you have a long wait ahead before the arrival of help, a drink may be beneficial.

These general directions apply in most cases, but there are certain kinds of bleeding which either need particular attention, or which may be a sign of serious internal injuries requiring urgent expert attention.

From the Scalp

Scalp wounds often cause heavy bleeding, but you should be very careful when examining bleeding from this area not to press too hard or probe the wound in case there is a fracture of the skull underneath. Act as follows:

1. Apply direct moderate pressure with a pad as already described until acute bleeding has stopped.

2. Find a dressing larger than the wound itself, or make one, and bandage it firmly in place, using the crepe bandage from the kit.

3. If there is a foreign body, such as a stone, embedded in the wound, find the scissors and cut a hole in the centre of a dressing. Place this over the wound so that the projecting object can poke through the hole. Never put a bandage over a wound with something sticking out of it, because the pressure of the bandage could drive the object further into the wound, and in the case of the skull could cause serious injury.

From the Ear

Pay special attention to this because such bleeding may indicate a head injury. Blood or a discharge of straw-coloured fluid from the ear could indicate a fracture at the base of the skull. If you find such a discharge, place a dressing or pad over the ear and secure it lightly in position with tape. If it is possible to move the casualty very gently without disturbing him too much, lay him down with his head slightly inclined towards the injured side. But if he is unconscious, leave him where he is unless he is in serious danger. Don't try to plug the ear with anything to stop the discharge. Get help as a matter of urgency.

From the Nose

Nosebleeds occur very frequently and do not really constitute an emergency, but they can continue for a long period of time unless you know how to stop them. Although not dangerous for short periods, they are inconvenient and annoying to have to cope with on a day out walking or climbing. However, it is quite simple to control a nose-bleed:

1. Make the casualty sit on the ground with his head slightly forward. Check that he is breathing through his mouth.
2. Pinch the soft part of the nose between your finger and thumb gently for about ten minutes. Make sure that clothing round his neck and chest is loose.
3. When the bleeding stops, be careful not to make it start again. Tell the victim not to blow his nose because this will dislodge the blood clot which is controlling the bleeding.
4. If bleeding continues for some time, the victim should go to a doctor as soon as is practical when he returns. If bleeding persists, never try to plug the nostrils with tissues or cotton wool. Try to prevent the victim from swallowing his blood, or he may feel sick.

From the Palm

This warrants special mention because the palm of the hand is very well supplied with blood vessels, and a relatively minor injury can cause quite heavy bleeding. The palm often takes the brunt of a fall because it is often the first point of contact between the body and the ground, and then takes the full weight of the body. If you fall on rocky ground you may cut your palm quite badly. When dealing with a victim of this sort of injury, act as follows:

1. Press a sterile dressing firmly over the wound and hold it in place until the bleeding stops.
2. If you are certain that there is no fracture to the arm in addition to the cut, lift the arm and hold it slightly raised.
3. To keep the dressing in place, bend the victim's fingers over it, as if he were clenching his fist. Then bandage the fingers firmly with a folded triangular bandage, tying it across the knuckles.

4. Support the hand and arm by resting them in a triangular sling.

5. If there is a sharp object like a stone embedded in the wound, or if you think that the arm or wrist may be broken, control the bleeding in the usual way, and simply support the arm in a sling.

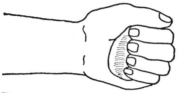

Fig. 16. Control of bleeding from the palm.

From a Varicose Vein

A varicose vein is a mass of bluish-black bulging veins visible under the skin, usually on the calf of the leg. These swollen blood vessels have their own reservoir of blood which, if punctured, can cause heavy bleeding. Varicose veins are the result of defective valves controlling blood flow and pressure and, while not dangerous in themselves, can cause problems if accidentally burst. If the right action is not taken quickly, a victim could bleed to death.

A minor fall can be enough to burst a varicose vein. If a varicose vein bursts, act immediately:

1. Press a sterile dressing and padding directly over the vein, and hold it in place.

2. As soon as practical, ask the victim to lie flat on his back, and then raise the affected leg in the air as high as you can. Meanwhile, keep the dressing held firmly in place and loosen any tight clothing above the vein, for example knee britches or garters.

3. Keep the leg raised until help arrives, even if this takes several hours. There is no need to hold it up all the time — either move the victim to a place where he can rest the leg

at a higher level than the rest of his body or build a support using a rucksack or a pile of stones.

4. Even if the bleeding stops, you may still need the assistance of a rescue team to help the casualty off the hills in case he has suffered from shock. However, if you are in such an isolated place that you have no alternative but to walk without help to safety, remember to check frequently that bleeding has not started again.

From a Miscarriage

This is not a common occurrence on the hills, because not many pregnant women undertake arduous walks or climbs; but it can happen, and indeed has happened. Whatever the other medical problems caused by miscarriage, or spontaneous abortion, the first is bleeding, possibly severe bleeding, especially if it is caused by a heavy fall or injury. Miscarriage can also occur early in pregnancy, when the victim is not yet aware she is pregnant; the most likely time is the third or fourth month. If it should happen within your group, act as follows:

1. Prevent the casualty from walking any further and make her lie down as quietly as possible until help arrives. There may still be a chance of saving the baby, but movement of the mother could worsen matters and destroy any hopes of the pregnancy continuing normally.

2. Do whatever you can to lessen the effects of shock and pain, and keep the victim as warm and comfortable as possible. Send for help.

BLISTERS

Blisters are minor inconveniences causing major misery. They can transform a happy day on the hills to a painful slog. Although a relatively trivial complaint they produce a great amount of suffering.

When Are They Likely to Happen?

Blisters are most likely to form on the feet and ankles if boots are too tight, or new and stiff, or ill-fitting in any other way. Victims are often occasional walkers or climbers, whose boots are not often worn and whose feet are unaccustomed to this type of heavier footwear. Sometimes nylon socks worn next to the skin aggravate the problem by failing to absorb sweat.

What Happens When They Form?

When a boot and sock are rubbing uncomfortably against the skin, they cause a friction which damages the little blood vessels just under the skin, causing small amounts of plasma to leak from the vessels. This fluid collects under the skin and if left alone would in time disperse on its own, as long as no further pressure was put on the area. But if the victim continues to walk so that the blister becomes more and more uncomfortable, the skin holding the fluid will break, allowing it to escape, and also letting germs in. In time, the affected area will become an open sore if nothing is done to stop the friction.

What Can I Do?

The big question is: To pop or not to pop? Normally, it would probably be better to leave nature to heal the blister without interfering. But if you are on the hills when the blister forms, you will have to live with it until you reach home again. So you must not only treat the blister and prevent it from getting worse, but also make it possible for the victim to continue the walk with as little discomfort as possible. This means not simply easing the pain. Blisters are an annoying distraction, and not only rob the victim of his general enjoyment, but can also reduce his powers of concentration. There is always the danger that, if a small blister becomes a preoccupation, the victim may become careless and place himself in danger. However, to ease his pain sufficiently to enable him to continue walking normally, do as follows:

1. At the first sign of any discomfort, before a blister has the chance to form, cover the sore area with a dressing and tape from the first-aid kit, so that the blister cannot form and the dressing can act as a protective pad to prevent friction.

2. If it is too late and a blister has already formed, you can pop it with a sterile pin, needle or sharp blade. For many people, this may seem to be breaking a golden rule, because traditionally most of us were taught never to pop blisters. But if you don't release the fluid and the victim continues walking, as he has to, the blister will pop on its own and will be much more painful. There will also be a higher risk of infection. Instead, you can anticipate nature. Hold a pin or needle or sharp blade in a flame until red hot, or sterilize it by boiling it for three minutes, and then gently prick the edge of the blister so that the fluid can drain away. Then cover the area with a sterile dressing and keep it in place with tape, or with a bandage which will also act as padding to prevent further friction.

Avoid blisters by wearing two pairs of socks, or one pair and one pair of woollen stockings, and never wear nylon socks next to the skin because they do not absorb the sweat from the foot and can soon soften the skin. If your boots are new, or if you do not wear them often, try to break them in at home by wearing them in the garden or while taking the dog for a walk. When you buy a pair of boots, make sure they are not too tight. Apart from causing the formation of blisters, tight boots can be dangerous if they impede circulation, especially in very cold weather when the result can be frostbite or frostnip.

BROKEN BONES
SEE FRACTURES, page 103.

BURNS

Emergency Action Quick Reference (Major Burns)

1. Check that there is no breathing difficulty and that the heart has not stopped. If either is the case refer to mouth-to-mouth assisted breathing (page 59) and cardiac massage (page 62).
2. Check for shock (page 153) and treat if necessary.
3. Immerse burnt part immediately in clean cold water for ten minutes, without removing any charred clothing which may be stuck to the skin. If sufficient cold water for immersion is not available, cover with water-soaked padding.
4. Clean wound with water and cover with thick dry dressing.

What Are They?

Burns are areas of damaged tissue caused by skin contact with flame, boiling water or other sources of heat, electric currents, acids and other corrosive poisons. Not only can the damaged tissue constitute serious injury, but burns cause blood vessels to leak plasma, the fluid part of blood, and if this leakage is serious it may cause problems in blood circulation round the body, which is the basis of shock. So if you are confronted with a bad burn, you must pay as much attention to the effects of shock as to the burn itself. The shock can be fatal even though the burn may not.

Most of us associate burns with cooking and hot fat, or careless firework handling, or serious road crashes, and few people would find an obvious link between burns and hill-walking to justify their inclusion in mountain first aid. Yet every year rescue teams come across cases of quite severe burns on the hills, due to several commonly occurring accidents. One of the easiest things to do with a primus stove balanced precariously on rough ground on a hillside is to knock it over, and many burns are the result of this sort of accident. Victims are injured by the stove and also by the spillage of whatever was being cooked over it. The fuel for the stove brings its own problems. Not only are gas canisters by themselves extremely volatile potential bombs, but campers continue to use their stoves in very small confined areas inside their tents, and even change cylinders in the tent. Campers who use stoves for heating or cooking inside their tents face a high risk of fire, should the heater get knocked over and waste gas ignite. Tent fires are quite common, and even if the victims escape alive and uninjured their camping gear and personal luggage doesn't usually come off quite so well.

Another danger involves suffocation by fumes from a stove inside the tent, should there be inadequate ventilation. Burns on the hills have also been caused by rope friction, and even by careless handling of distress flares. Of course, these examples do not amount to a major mountain hazard, and with vigilance most of them can be avoided.

How to Recognize a Burn

Identifying a burn is much easier than trying to locate hidden injuries or discover why a person has suddenly become ill. Skin in contact with great heat or acid produces a burn. If you are with the victim, you will probably be aware that an accident has happened.

The difference between major and minor burns is the area of the body damaged. If it covers more than 15 per cent of the body's surface, the burn is major.

Minor Burns

A minor burn may simply form a blister, and need no special first aid beyond helping to lessen the pain and comforting the victim. However, even minor burns can be deep and break the skin, so be on the lookout for shock, especially if the victim looks very pale or feels faint, and treat accordingly. Treat the wound as for a major burn.

Major Burns

In cases of major burns a large area will be affected, the skin may be broken and the area of the burn will look raw and red. There will be great pain initially unless the burn is so deep that nerve endings have been destroyed, and there may be breathing difficulty and shock.

What Can I Do?

1. The treatment for major and minor burn wounds is the same, but with major burns, shock and breathing problems, if present, must be treated quickly (see the sections on shock (pages 153–7) and mouth-to-mouth assisted breathing (pages 59–61)). The burn wound should then be treated with clean, cold water, preferably by immersion for ten minutes. There may be some water near by which can be carried to the victim in containers such as billy cans or polythene exposure bags. Small burnt areas can then be immersed. For large areas, this may not be possible, and the best alternative is to cover them with water-soaked padding. Never use stagnant water, as infection can quickly occur in an open burn wound. If no fast-running water is available, or there is no water at all, it is preferable simply to exclude air by covering the burn with a dry sterile dressing.

2. Pain-killing tablets can be given, which will also assist in reducing shock.

3. Remove any charred clothing after immersion or soaking, and clean the wound gently with clean water.

4. Cover the wound thickly with dry dressings to absorb the plasma which will seep from it and otherwise form a crust. The dressing will require additional padding if the seepage soaks through.

5. NEVER smear any cream or greasy or oil-based ointment over the burn. This could dry to a hard crust on

top of the burn which will result in further injury and pain when removed. If you are not sure what to do about a burn, do nothing beyond helping reduce shock, which is a more dangerous threat to life than the burn itself. In this case, kindness and reassurance that anyone can give by way of comfort can actually help to save life.

Should I Send for Help?

Yes, unless the burn is minor, because the damage underlying even small areas of burn may be quite serious and cause sudden shock. Judge the condition of the victim to help you distinguish between a minor incident and an accident in which you need experienced help.

Can I Give a Drink?

Yes. The effect of a cup of warm tea or coffee can do wonders in controlling shock. In the case of serious burns a drink can also help to restore fluid lost through damaged blood vessels.

It is far easier to prevent burns than to treat them. Make sure that portable stoves are securely positioned and not likely to blow over in a gust of wind. Don't use them inside tents unless they are well ventilated, and even then avoid doing so unless it is impossible to cook outside. Never change a gas cylinder inside a tent. If anything catches fire, don't try to smother the flames with inflammable materials such as nylon anoraks or sleeping bags. Use either water or any non-inflammable material available.

CHEST INJURY

Emergency Action Quick Reference

1. In the case of visible 'sucking' wound, seal the wound with a sterile dressing and tape to prevent further escape of air from the chest wall.

2. Ensure the victim's airway is clear (see page 58).

3. Turn him on his injured side and send for help.

4. If breathing difficulty persists, and yet there is no sign of a puncture of the chest wall, feel gently for broken ribs. Lay the victim on his injured side and send for help.

Certain chest injuries are as serious, and as likely to be fatal, as some head injuries if not dealt with promptly. The 'sucking' wound chest injury is caused when something hard or sharp penetrates the chest wall and the lung collapses. Air is then sucked in through the hole in the chest instead of through the mouth, but it cannot escape because the wound acts as a one-way valve. The lung remains inactive, air builds up in the chest, and the victim becomes short of oxygen and cannot breathe. Unless the hole is temporarily patched up immediately, thus restoring a vacuum within the chest, the victim may not survive.

Broken ribs can also cause breathing difficulty when the bones form an obstacle which moves in the opposite direction to the rest of the chest wall. When the victim breathes in, the broken bone mass is sucked in just when the chest should be expanding; and when he breathes out, the bone obstruction is blown outwards when the chest should be deflating. This makes breathing very difficult and the victim soon becomes short of oxygen. If he panics, his struggle to breathe will make matters worse. You may also notice frothy blood coming out of his mouth which may indicate that a broken rib has punctured a lung.

When Are They Most Likely to Happen?

'Sucking' wound injuries are more common in climbing accidents, because they are normally caused by a heavy fall onto sharp rock, or something pointed like an ice axe. A chest injury caused by several broken ribs could, however, be the result of an accident as simple as a heavy fall while climbing over a gate or wall.

What Should I Notice?

One of the first signs of a chest injury will be a bluish colour in the face, especially around the lips, which is caused by oxygen starvation if breathing becomes difficult. If you notice this bluish tinge after an accident involving the chest, check immediately to see if breathing is normal. Look at the chest and listen. Breathing may be irregular or shallow, and you may hear a hissing sound if air is escaping through a puncture in the chest wall, or a sucking sound if it is entering the chest through the wound. If no visible damage is present but you suspect that broken ribs may be causing the breathing difficulty, especially if you see any sign of blood coming from the mouth, feel very gently with the flat of your hand for any part of the chest wall which has become separated and may be moving in reverse to the chest as the victim struggles to breathe in and out.

What Can I Do?

In the case of an obvious sucking wound, act at once:

1. Make sure first of all that the breathing difficulty is not being made worse by airway blockage (see page 58). Clear any obstruction.

2. When you have checked that the airway is clear, use a sterile dressing from the first-aid kit and tape it over the wound with plaster.

3. Turn the victim on his injured side so that his lungs

can drain more easily if necessary, and so that his own weight will keep the seal firmly in place over the wound. This position will also ensure that any broken ribs or separated part of the chest wall are held in place by the victim's weight.

If there is no chest wound but breathing difficulty persists, act as follows:

1. Reassure the victim and prevent him from panicking as he tries to breathe.

2. Suspect that breathing is being made difficult by the action of broken ribs within the rib cage and feel gently with your hand to find any abnormality.

3. If you can locate any part of the chest wall which seems to have come adrift from the rest, press it gently with your hand to prevent it from moving in reverse to the rest of the chest. If breathing improves at once, strap a dressing over the area with a crepe bandage tied across the chest to hold it in place, and lay the victim with his weight pressing on the injured side.

4. Tell him to breathe deeply and encourage him to cough up any blood or spittle which may have become trapped in his lungs, to lessen the risk of infection later. In all cases of chest injury, send for help urgently.

Can I Give a Drink?

If particularly requested, a drink may be given in small sips.

CRAMP

Cramp occurs quite often on the hills and normally affects walkers in the thighs or calves. It is a painful, but not in itself serious, spasm of muscles often caused by a salt deficiency, following heavy perspiration. Other causes include narrowing of blood vessels, so that during brisk exercise insufficient amounts of blood flow to the legs. It can also result from poor muscular co-ordination in walkers who are unused to vigorous exercise, or from an awkward stride due to blisters or uncomfortable boots. Victims suffering from cramp complain of a sharp pain within the affected muscle and most people have either experienced this before, or have seen somebody else with it, and thus will probably recognize it immediately.

What Can I Do?

Cramp can easily be relieved, but can recur once it has started.

1. If the weather is hot and the victim has been sweating freely, you can help replace the salt that he has lost by giving him a drink of cold water, adding half a teaspoon of salt per pint. Encourage him to drink as much as he likes.

2. If the cramp is in the thigh, straighten the knee with both your hands. Then put one hand under the heel of the foot and raise the leg, while pressing the knee with your

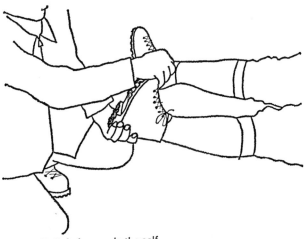

Fig. 17. Relief of cramp in the calf.

other hand downwards. The object of this is to stretch the affected muscle and relieve the spasm.

3. If the cramp is in the calf or foot, straighten the knee and push the heel down with one hand while forcibly pushing the toes up towards the shin with the other hand. This should effectively stretch the cramped muscle.

4. When the victim recovers, abandon plans for the rest of the day's activities and concentrate only on helping the victim down to safety. Cramp may recur if you continue exercise under the conditions which caused it before, and continuous cramp could result in complete immobilization, in which case you will need help to carry the victim off the hill.

DIABETES

General

Diabetes is a disease which affects the way in which we convert glucose into energy. Natural insulin normally brings about this conversion, but if the natural supply is deficient it has to be supplemented. The dosage of extra insulin has to be accurate, otherwise things start to go wrong.

Most diabetics understand their own condition so well that they manage to live perfectly normal lives as long as they eat at regular times and keep the delicate balance between their blood–sugar levels and the extra amounts of insulin they have to give themselves to help convert sugar into energy. Everyday life does not usually present them with any problems that they cannot deal with promptly themselves, but if they take part in activities that they are not used to in conditions which may not be as regular and controlled as life is at home, they may become ill, and need very rapid help from someone who understands what may have gone wrong. Hill-walking and climbing can impose those extra physical strains and you should be aware of the danger signs so that you can correct the imbalance

immediately. This knowledge could also prove useful elsewhere.

By far the commonest sort of imbalance is caused when a
diabetic has an excess of insulin left over after he has used
up all his supplies of sugar, and this is the condition encountered most frequently. The diabetic walker takes his
normal dose of insulin, eats a normal breakfast and then
may use abnormally large amounts of glucose owing to his
unaccustomed exercise. His supplies of sugar to balance the
insulin are used up too quickly, and this can be further
aggravated if he does not eat a properly balanced meal at
his regular time. This is likely to happen if he is with a party
who do not stop to eat, or if he loses track of time. He will
then suddenly suffer what is called an 'insulin reaction'.
Fortunately this has such characteristic symptoms that you
can guess what has happened very quickly and put it right.

However, there is another complication of diabetes
which, while it occurs less frequently, will eventually result
in coma and subsequent death if it is untreated. Its onset is
much slower than the instant insulin reaction, so even if
you are in a very remote place there will probably be time
to get help before the situation has become too dangerous.
The symptoms of a diabetic coma are the complete opposite
of the signs which indicate an insulin reaction; but the first
aid is the same for both: you treat the condition as though
it were an insulin reaction, because it probably is; but if it
is not, then what you have done can in time be corrected
and not cause undue harm.

Insulin Reaction

This is dealt with first, as it is by far the most probable cause
of the trouble.

When Is It Likely to Happen?

The reaction occurs when the insulin burns up the sugar
too quickly, so that the body runs out of glucose. Energetic

exercise of the type involved in hill-walking or climbing, especially in cold weather, uses up energy very rapidly, and if it is not replaced by means of food a diabetic will soon feel the ill effects of this lack of sugar and excess of insulin.

What Happens When a Diabetic Has an Insulin Reaction?

The first sign noticed by the diabetic is usually a feeling of mild hunger. Then he starts to sweat, feels dizzy and goes very pale, and his skin feels moist to touch. By this stage, he usually recognizes what is happening to him. If no action is taken, he will breathe very shallowly, tremble, have double or blurred vision and start to become mentally confused, often displaying extraordinary behaviour, like trying to undress or being abnormally bad-tempered and aggressive. Finally he loses consciousness.

What Can I Do?

1. You can reverse these symptoms dramatically at any point before the unconscious collapse by giving the diabetic something with sugar in it, for example a sugar lump, sweet, chocolate or a sweet drink. Within 30 seconds to a minute, the signs will disappear completely, and the diabetic may not even remember what has happened. Often diabetics carry their own emergency supply of sugar in their pockets, so, if you have none easily available, check in the victim's pockets or rucksack for sweets or sugar.

2. Don't give too much sugar too quickly, or the diabetic will feel sick. Two sugar lumps, or the equivalent, will be sufficient, and after he has recovered he should have his meal or snack before continuing.

3. If the diabetic does not respond to the sugar, or if he is unconscious when you find him and you cannot give him sugar, go for help urgently.

4. If you are with someone whom you know to be a diabetic, give him sugar at the first sign of *any* illness, even if it turns out not to have been an insulin reaction. The

first-aid rule is: always regard the symptoms as reaction, and act immediately. You can find out later if you were correct. If you were not, little harm will have been done.

5. If ever you should find somebody who is obviously ill but with no apparent cause, and who is unable to tell you why he is ill, such as a reaction victim by the time he has become mentally confused, you should always check his pockets or wrist for a sign of identification. Most diabetics wear Medic-Alert bracelets or some similar means of identification in case of illness. If you do find such a badge on anybody who has been taken ill suddenly, always treat them first as though they have an insulin reaction by giving sugar.

Diabetic Coma

This is, in every way, the complete opposite of insulin reaction, because it is caused by an insufficient quantity of insulin in the body rather than excess. It has its own particular set of symptoms, but it is much slower to develop than reaction, and is very unusual in careful diabetics.

When Is It Likely to Happen?

It happens most commonly if a diabetic forgets to take a regular dose of insulin, or if he is preoccupied, gives himself too little or thinks that he has taken the dose when he has not. It can also occur if he is ill or injured, or when his normal balance is upset by some other external factor. The more serious the injury, the greater the disturbance and possibility that coma will follow. But without the proper chemical tests on his blood–sugar level, it is impossible to be certain that the diabetic is suffering from the onset of coma, and the most you can do is to be aware of the physical symptoms.

What Happens When a Diabetic Is Threatened by Coma?

The signs will be seen only very gradually. The diabetic is not hungry, as in reaction, but very thirsty and has to pass water frequently. His skin will feel dry and hot, but he will not be dizzy. His breathing becomes very slow and laboured, and you will notice a distinctive fruity smell to his breath. He will become very drowsy and lethargic.

What Can I Do?

1. Give him a lump of sugar in case he is suffering from insulin reaction and the symptoms are not clear. You must rule out this possibility rapidly before considering anything else.

2. If the diabetic understands what is happening, he may know that he needs more insulin, and if that has happened before he is probably carrying a supply with him. In this case, he can treat himself. If he has no extra supplies, or if he has forgotten to bring a regular dose with him, or if he is out on the hills for longer than he had anticipated, then send for help urgently with an accurate message describing what has occurred and what the diabetic tells you that he needs, so that a rescue party can bring the necessary insulin.

3. Make the diabetic rest completely. On no account should he try and walk to safety himself. Be calm and reassuring until help arrives.

There is no reason at all why a fit diabetic should not enjoy walking and climbing, but if he is in a group he should inform the group leader that he is a diabetic and what action can be taken to help him if he is unwell. If you are walking in a small group with a diabetic friend, make sure that he understands his particular needs and also that he is carrying an identity card with details of the condition and necessary units of insulin in case he should become isolated from the main party, or even knocked unconscious in an accident. Make sure also that he knows how to treat himself, especially if he is young and normally under parental supervision. Check that he is carrying his own supplies of extra sugar, or insulin, or both. If there is any doubt about the timing of the walk or climb, the diabetic must allow for this. In very remote places when the planned route is isolated and very far from help, he should carry a couple of days' supply of insulin in case the party become lost. He should also carry the right quantities of food for himself, and be responsible for eating at the right time.

DROWNING

Emergency Action Quick Reference

1. If the victim has stopped breathing, check that his airway is clear (see page 58) before attempting resuscitation.

2. Begin mouth-to-mouth assisted breathing (see page 59) and cardiac massage (see page 62) if necessary, and continue until he recovers or his muscles stiffen as rigor mortis sets in after death.

3. If he recovers, lay him on his side so that his lungs can drain without danger of his choking.

4. Send for help, and protect the victim from the cold.

The clear fresh water of mountain lakes and streams is a most inviting sight on a hot summer's day to a walker or climber; however, some would-be swimmers do not realize that such waters have their own particular dangers, and in recent years there have been several cases of death by drowning on the hills.

Some mountain tarns are very deep, and while water near the surface can be quite warm, a swimmer may suddenly find himself in an area of very cold water and become paralysed with cramp caused by extreme change in temperature. Others take to the deep water on full stomachs and develop cramp. Swimmers also fail to appreciate that swift and forceful mountain streams can easily sweep them to their deaths. Incidents have also occurred during attempts to cross fast-flowing streams in full winter flood. But drowning is not the only danger; the bottom of still tarns where there is little movement of water to erode and smooth the bed can cause quite serious injuries if swimmers and divers come into contact with the sharp stones which may lie hidden, and such injuries can also contribute to drowning. It is therefore important for hill walkers and climbers to know what should be done in the event of swimming accidents.

What Happens When a Victim Is Drowning?

Drowning is suffocation by water and death is caused by a sudden imbalance in body fluid. The lungs fill with water, which displaces air, so that the victim cannot breathe. The fresh water is absorbed through the lung walls into the bloodstream, which it rapidly dilutes, upsetting the balance of all the vital substances in the blood, and the victim dies. However, there are cases when the victim chokes to death before even swallowing any water when he is in danger of drowning. A reflex action to prevent the entry of water into the lungs causes the larynx to constrict, and the victim starts to choke. Fortunately, when he loses consciousness, after breathing stops, the muscles relax and if assisted breathing is given at once his life can be saved.

What Can I Do?

1. As soon as the victim is dragged to the safety of dry land, lay him on his side if he is still breathing so that he can drain his lungs more easily of any water he has swallowed without choking or inhaling his own vomit.

2. If breathing has stopped, it is most important to clear his airway before starting assisted breathing (see page 58).

Apart from the obvious danger that his tongue may be blocking his airway, he may also be choking on anything he may have swallowed, for example strands of water weed.

3. Once the airway is clear, proceed as directed on pages 59–61, making quite sure that the victim is in the correct recovery position on his side after breathing restarts, to prevent him from drowning in his own secretions after the initial danger is past. If he fails to recover at once, do not give up but continue artificial resuscitation. It may be some time before you succeed and you may have to go on for up to an hour.

4. Send for help urgently. If the victim is recovering, prevent him from becoming cold in his wet and shocked state. Hypothermia can develop rapidly in these circumstances, so insulate the casualty from the ground if he is still lying in the recovery position, and cover him with spare clothing.

EXPOSURE
SEE HYPOTHERMIA, pages 134–44.

FATIGUE

Fatigue is one of the most interesting problems experienced on the hills, and there is much more to it than just sitting down and feeling tired. A victim can suffer extreme tiredness, and then suddenly energy returns. Very few people can explain the fascinating process of getting a second wind and finishing the day's walking or climbing with vigour after a period of great fatigue. Although fatigue can be defined in terms of muscle tiredness, there seems to be a strong link between the extent of tiredness and the enjoyment, or dislike, of the pursuit.

Many walkers who enjoy the challenge of an all-day scramble on the hills go home with little more than stiff muscles and pleasant, relaxing tiredness, even if they are unused to such exercise. However, others develop signs of fatigue quite quickly and give up the planned route. Although there is no definite scientific evidence, it does seem clear that the more a walker enjoys what he is doing and actively wants to do it, the less chance there is that he will become over-tired. People who are not so strongly motivated to enjoy the hills, for example, school children in parties who have had no choice whether or not they take part in an expedition or who may not know by previous experience exactly what is involved, seem much more likely to be victims of fatigue.

The problem of fatigue is that the victim is not only uncomfortable and distressed, but also far more susceptible to such dangers as hypothermia than someone who is coping well with the exertion. So, once you recognize the signs of fatigue, you must be careful to take them seriously as a first-aider, before more dangerous conditions develop.

What Can I Do?

1. Let the victim rest, and give him something to eat or drink to help increase his energy.

2. Instead of showing annoyance and impatience that the victim is slowing the party down, give him plenty of reassurance and restore confidence in himself. The tiredness may be some sort of reaction to fears of being unable to keep up or finish the day's programme.

3. Don't let the victim worry about his own tiredness, and don't let him lose all enjoyment in what he is doing. Give him some sort of small goal which he can aim for, to restore his motivation; it need be only a rest and a snack every half hour. After he has shown signs of abnormal stress and tiredness, continue stopping through the day at regular intervals to let him rest.

4. If the victim does not respond to food and rest, and could be in danger of hypothermia, forget your plans for the day and return to safety. There may be more to it than just

tiredness, and the victim should be helped down before fatigue becomes illness.

5. Even if things are going wrong, and you are lost or benighted or very cold, remember the importance of keeping morale high. Low morale is a key factor in the onset of hypothermia and state of mind is a vital factor in fighting physical illness and injury.

FITS AND SEIZURES

Every year in Britain, there are several recorded cases of walkers and climbers suffering from fits on the hills, although nobody quite knows why fits should be quite so common there. The sight of a friend or fellow-walker having a fit is very alarming, but it need not be if you understand a little of what is happening and what you can do to prevent any further mishap, though there is nothing anyone can do to prevent the fit itself.

A fit is caused by abnormal activity in the brain which results in interference with sensations, movements and often consciousness. Experts now think that fits are often caused by certain other conditions, but for hundreds of years fits of the epileptic type have been the subject of fear and superstition, with associations of possession by the devil. If you see somebody suffering a fit, forget all the old wives' tales you may have heard and don't be frightened by his or her uncontrolled movements. Instead, you can make a series of basic checks as part of your first aid which could be of some practical help to the victim.

When Is a Fit Likely to Happen?

If anybody knew the answer to this question, he would probably be able to tell the world exactly why some people have fits. They are unpredictable, and there is nothing that an untrained person can notice about the victim until he has actually started having the fit. Even if you knew when it was coming, you could not prevent it. Sometimes victims will recognize their own particular symptoms and danger signals. Fits have also been known to strike victims of head injuries.

What Do They Look Like?

There are two sorts of fits. One is very minor, the other more serious, but neither is difficult to recognize. The minor sort, often experienced by children, is just a few moments of unconsciousness, after which victims often do not remember what has happened. A major fit is more dramatic. The victim often falls unconscious, sometimes with a sort of cry, and his muscles become quite stiff and then start to twitch violently. His movements are uncontrolled and if left un-aided he may bite his tongue. Sometimes the victim empties his bladder, and the wild movements and violence of the spasms may go on for as long as two minutes or so. After it is all over, some victims recover by going into a deep sleep or trance, while others may behave in rather odd and un-characteristic ways.

Although the fit is a most upsetting experience for the victim, if he is aware of what is happening, the main hazard is that of the injuries which may result if he is in a dangerous place, such as a crag or steep slope, when it occurs. In addition, he may choke himself during the fit or afterwards if he is unconscious. The correct first aid is to try and lessen these dangers for him; the fit itself is beyond your control, or his.

What Should I Do?

Once you have realized that someone is having a fit, act as follows:

1. If the fit occurs in a steep or rocky place, don't let the victim roll or fall, and try to prevent any collision with sharp rocks or boulders.

2. Restrain the victim as far as is possible without undue force. Total restraint will not be possible.

3. Loosen any tight clothing that you can reach, for example an anorak hood tied under his chin which may restrict his neck dangerously.

4. If the victim is going blue in the face, he is having breathing difficulty. The probable cause of this is airway block by the tongue. This can be difficult to deal with because in a fit the victim often has tightly clenched teeth You will have to force them open by means of a spoon or similar object wrapped in a handkerchief. Once the mouth is opened, wedge it open with the handkerchief-covered instrument, and deal with the airway block as described under assisted breathing (page 58).

5. If breathing has actually stopped, the victim will no longer be in a fit, so resuscitation will be relatively easy.

6. Once the fit is over, be ready with basic first-aid comfort, warmth and reassurance. If the fit has been very minor, the victim may feel that he can walk down without help, but, if he does, be prepared in case another fit occurs. If the fit has been a major one, you will have to go for help, and, if you are in any doubt at all about what to do, get help rather than take a chance.

Can I Give a Drink?

Once the fit is over, you can give a drink slowly, in small sips, but watch all the time to make sure that the victim is fully conscious and does not choke.

FOOD POISONING

It can be very alarming if, when you are miles from the nearest road or house, a companion suddenly doubles up with stomach pains and starts to vomit or have diarrhoea. This sort of illness is very difficult to treat. The victim starts to weaken quite soon and often collapses eventually, so that the journey to safety has to be assisted by rescuers. Although you cannot be certain, the problem may well be caused by some sort of food poisoning, which can strike the victim hours after the infected food is eaten.

What Can I Do?

When a companion is taken ill in this way, you can do very little except to get help if the person becomes too ill to walk down alone. If help is a long time in coming (maybe as long as several hours away) and the victim is very sick, you will have to try to prevent him from becoming too dehydrated. If you have any drinking water, or if there is drinkable water available, give the victim frequent drinks, even if he continues to vomit. Nothing more can be done until the victim reaches safety and a proper diagnosis of the trouble can be made.

If you suspect that anyone has just eaten poisonous plants, berries or fungi, waste no time waiting to see what will happen. Make the person vomit immediately by sticking a finger, yours or his, down the back of his throat, or give him salty water to drink. The object is to make him as sick as you can as quickly as possible so that the poison can be vomited before it reaches the blood stream. If you can possibly preserve a little of the vomited matter in a plastic bag or tin lid, this may help to identify the poison so that the right antidote can be given more rapidly.

FOREIGN OBJECTS IN THE EYE

The natural watering of the eye is often all that is needed to wash out a foreign body, and relief comes at once. But on the hills it may not be quite so easily dealt with. A high wind, for instance, can propel an object such as an insect or particle of grit into the eye with some force, making removal difficult. Walking on scree can also cause eye trouble. The scree is made up of tiny fragments of rock; some of it is small enough to be blown into the eye in a strong wind, or there may be someone walking above the victim sending down little showers of stone and dust. What may begin as a very minor irritation could end up as a major problem if the wrong first aid is carried out.

What Happens When Something Gets in the Eye?

The foreign object immediately causes the eye to secrete tears, and if this doesn't wash the object out of the eye the tears will prevent the victim from being able to see where he is going, so he will have to stop. If the object is soft, like a small, squashy insect, it may be possible for the first-aider to remove it very gently with a finger or the corner of a handkerchief. But if the object is hard, like grit of some sort, any attempt to poke it out by these means may simply drag the object across the cornea, which is the circular window in the front of the eye behind which are the iris (coloured) and pupil (appears black). If the cornea is scratched or scarred, ulcers can develop later and ultimately that eye can go blind. The link between the tiny foreign object causing minor discomfort and future blindness may seem rather remote, but misguided first-aid attempts to remove sharp intruders from the eye have actually ended in blindness. It isn't always impossible to help a victim with something in his eye, but there are times when first aid can be very harmful. One day you may have to judge whether to have a go at removing the trouble, or leave well alone.

What Can I Do?

1. Find somewhere sheltered, so that the force of the wind doesn't make the eye water even more, and stop the victim rubbing the affected eye or poking it. If the object is not easily visible, very gently pull the eyelid away from the eye so that you can see inside, and pull the skin back from under the eyelashes to have a look at the lower part of the eye. Sometimes this action alone will be enough to dislodge the

object from under the eyelid, or wherever it has become trapped.

2. If you can see what the object is, decide whether it is likely to be sharp or soft. The victim himself may be able to

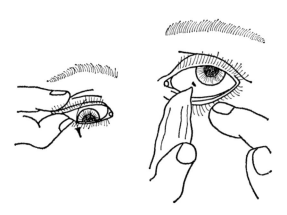

Fig. 18. Removal of foreign body from the eye.

tell you if it is hard or not from what he can feel. If, and only if, you are certain that it is something soft, and if you can move it without dragging it across or poking it into the centre of the eye, make a little point out of the corner of a clean handkerchief and very gently trap the object so that it stays on the handkerchief, and then remove it.

3. If the speck looks like grit or a small stone, or even a hard little bug or insect, leave it where it is and don't try to remove it, or the grit could scratch the cornea. Even if the victim complains that he won't be able to see, this is a far better state of affairs for him than a damaged cornea. Well-meaning friends may suggest poking at the eye with a matchstick covered with cotton wool, or other sharp-pointed small objects like orange sticks. Ignore their advice and offers of help. To get the stone or grit out, it may be

necessary to freeze the eye. This is certainly not a job for a first-aider on the hill.

4. If you cannot safely remove the object, or think it better not to try, go to the first-aid kit and find a sterile dressing and bandage. Make an eye patch to cover and close the affected eye, with a soft padding in the centre. This will relieve some of the victim's discomfort and pain as he tries to walk along and see the path through the irritated eye. Take the victim to a doctor or hospital as soon as you reach safety.

FRACTURES

General

A fracture is a broken bone. In most healthy people, bones are very strong and don't break easily, but thinner bones can be broken by a direct blow, and even the stronger ones can be broken by violent impact. If a bone is broken, it is often snapped in two completely. Fractures are common occurrences on the hills because the terrain increases the chances and dangers of a slip or fall. A tumble over a kerb edge or a fall on a city pavement may result in little worse than bruising, shock and sprain but the same fall on rough stony ground can be very much more harmful.

First aid for fractures mainly involves immobilization of the broken limb, to prevent further pain caused by movement at the point of the breakage. This is not difficult if you have received instruction and watched demonstrations of the techniques – but not so easy if you are doing it for the first time and from a book. So, although immobilization is accepted as a basic first-aid skill by most manuals, it may be advisable for anybody alone, untrained or lacking in confidence not to attempt it if expert help will soon be available, and simply to stick to the basics which are no less essential. After all, the victim could die of exposure if you fail to keep him warm and sheltered, but he is unlikely to die if you cannot tie the right bandages for a few hours.

There are several different kinds of fracture, some more serious than others.

The *simple*, or closed, fracture, is a break in a bone which does not cause the surface of the skin to be broken. This is usually more simple to deal with because it doesn't carry the added problems of controlling external bleeding as well as making the broken limb more comfortable.

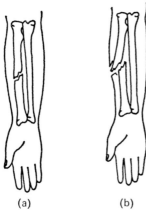

(a)   (b)

Fig. 19. Types of fracture : (a) Simple ; (b) Compound.

The *compound*, or open fracture, is more serious because the bone breaks in such a way as to puncture the skin, causing a nasty wound through which bacteria can enter and cause infection to the broken bone.

The *complicated* fracture is just what it says it is – complicated, especially for the first-aider. It is a break in a bone where the broken ends injure other organs, nerves or blood vessels, causing internal bleeding.

What Should I Notice?

The commonest causes of fracture are heavy falls on hard rock or wet grass, and you can suspect fractures after any such fall. If you are near the victim, you may even hear the snapping sound of a bone as it breaks. If the casualty is conscious, he will be in pain and will be able to indicate the point of the injury. Fractures are followed very quickly by swelling, and later by bruising. If the fracture is open, there will also be bleeding, which can be quite severe. The swelling can be considerable and may make removal of clothing painful and difficult. It will probably be necessary to remove clothing to investigate the extent of the injury and it may be less painful to cut it. Look for signs of swelling and deformity, which are clear indications of possible fracture – for example, in fracture of the femur, or thigh bone, the broken leg will sometimes appear shorter than the other because muscular contraction pulls at the two separate parts of the break. In many cases, however, it may be quite impossible without X-ray equipment to tell whether a bone is broken, dislocated or just cracked, or a ligament sprained. Faced with this uncertainty, always treat the injury as though it were a fracture. This may help to avoid causing further damage.

In an unconscious victim, examination should be more thorough, since fractures do not always occur at the obvious place. Falls onto an outstretched hand can cause arm and collar-bone breaks, for instance, and a fall caused by a foot which becomes tightly wedged between rocks can cause a break in the shin bone. However, if the victim is unconscious, discovering possible fractures is not the first priority, and before considering any broken bones full attention must be given to ensuring that the casualty continues to breathe without difficulty or airway blockage.

A conscious victim will usually be unable to move a fractured limb, but because this is not always the case, it is no sure test of whether the bone is broken.

What Can I Do?

Fractures are often combined with other more serious injuries if they result from a heavy fall. There may be breathing difficulty, bleeding and shock, which must all be treated urgently because they can result in death. Next in importance are the basic first-aid comforts of warmth, reassurance and shelter if necessary. These will help to reduce shock, lessen the risk of hypothermia in bad weather conditions, and help to prepare the victim for what may be a long wait until help arrives. Then you can attempt to treat the fracture itself: the main point is to relieve pain and prevent any further damage by immobilizing the fracture. Proceed as follows:

1. Don't move the victim unless it is necessary to prevent further injury. Other more serious injuries may be present, especially after a heavy fall.

2. Check that the victim is breathing without difficulty, and that his heart is beating. If not, start artificial resuscitation (see page 54).

3. Check for any bleeding, and stop it (see page 68).

4. Ensure the victim is sheltered and insulated from the cold to reduce shock, but do not overheat him.

5. If the victim is conscious, he will be able to indicate the source of pain. If he is not, feel carefully all over his body for signs of bleeding, swelling and deformity. You will probably need to remove his clothing. In order to minimize pain and damage, be very careful not to move the victim more than necessary. Use scissors to cut garments if it is easier.

6. Never move a conscious victim to another position if he indicates that he prefers to remain where he is. Ignore any text-book instructions advising the correct position for the injured limb, if they go against the victim's own natural inclinations – he is by far the best person to find the most comfortable position.

7. If the fracture prevents the victim from walking down unaided, or if he is suffering from shock, send for help. In certain cases, the victim may be able to make his own way to safety after immobilization of the limb.

Immobilization

In the case of an unconscious victim who is rolling around on the ground or jerking his body uncontrollably, it may be necessary to immobilize any fractures to prevent him from damaging himself further. However, in all other cases, unless you are confident that you can reduce the victim's

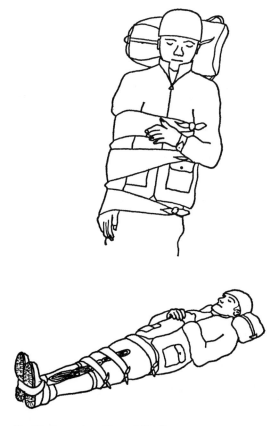

Fig. 20. Examples of immobilization.

pain by immobilization, it may be far better to do nothing and wait for help to arrive. The whole point of the technique is to prevent the movement of the injured limb and to protect it from being knocked or jolted, particularly during evacuation of the casualty. But if the victim is lying still, it is not essential to carry out this procedure until a rescue party arrives to move him. The victim will not suffer too much if you wait for experienced first-aiders to come and prepare the fracture for the journey down. Basically, immobilization involves securing the injured limb to the uninjured one to give it support, by means of padding and bandages. The finer details vary from fracture to fracture, but unfortunately it is quite easy to do it the wrong way. You may cause further deformity, or a failure in blood circulation if the bandages are tied too tightly, and the injured part swells. So, unless (*a*) immobilization is necessary to prevent further injury in an unconscious and restless victim; or (*b*) conditions dictate that you have to attempt your own rescue in a very remote place; or (*c*) the fracture is sited somewhere like the wrist and the victim intends to walk down unaided but with his arm secured to prevent jolting, generally it is better to wait for a rescue party to reach the accident scene with their experience and equipment rather than attempt immobilization yourself.

Certain specific fractures must now be dealt with individually.

Of the Skull

This is a very serious fracture, and there is very little you can do especially if it is accompanied by brain damage and unconsciousness (see Head Injuries, page 124).

When Might It Happen?

It can occur after a fall on the head, or a direct blow by something like a rock falling from above. A fracture at the base of the skull can result from falling heavily onto the feet or lower part of the spine, or by a hard blow on the lower jaw.

What Does It Look Like?

You may notice external injuries to the head, with bleeding and broken parts of the bone visible. You may also notice blood or a straw-coloured liquid coming from the ear or nose. The eyes may look bloodshot and gradually take on the appearance of a black eye.

What Can I Do?

1. Make sure that the casualty is breathing and that his airway is clear. If not, start assisted breathing as described on page 59.

2. Watch the pupils of both eyes and compare one with the other, keeping a record of what you see. This could be a very valuable guide for a doctor because it indicates what sort of damage may have happened to the brain.

3. Don't move the casualty. If there is a discharge from the ear, just place a sterile dressing over the ear lightly and turn the victim's head very gently so that that ear faces downwards.

Can I Give A Drink?

No.

Of the Ribs

A broken rib in itself is not serious but it may be accompanied by injuries to other organs such as the lungs, liver or spleen. If this happens, there could be extensive internal bleeding and difficulty in breathing.

When Might It Happen?

If the casualty falls heavily on his chest, or if he is hit in the ribs with a hard object like a falling stone, he is likely to break a rib or ribs.

What Does It Look Like?

If the fracture is under unbroken skin, it may not be visible, but there are other symptoms. The victim may have a very sharp pain near the injury, and it will probably hurt him to breathe deeply or cough. He may start to go blue and very breathless if the rib has injured his chest and lungs so badly that air is sucked out instead of into his lungs as he breathes. In such a case, refer to Chest Injury (see page 84).

What Can I Do?

1. If the fracture shows through the skin and looks very bad, do no more than control bleeding, and keep the casualty warm and reassured until help arrives.

2. If it seems to be a simple closed fracture of a rib, you could make the victim more comfortable by supporting the arm on the injured side in an arm sling if this seems to be the most comfortable position for him to hold the rib in place. However, let the victim decide if he wishes you to do this, otherwise wait for experienced help to arrive.

Can I Give a Drink?

Yes, but only in small amounts.

Of the Shoulders, Collar Bone, Arms and Wrists

Although a compound fracture of any of these is more difficult to treat than a closed break, fractures in these areas are generally less serious than those involving the skull or ribs, and certainly less incapacitating than fractures of the leg or ankle. As long as you are certain that there are no very serious underlying injuries, and provided that any bleeding and shock are controlled, it is usually possible for the victim to walk down the hill without assistance from a rescue team. Naturally, if he does not feel able or fit enough to tackle the walk down, never try to persuade him against his will – call for help rather than taking risks with other people's health. However, if you are in a very isolated place in bad conditions it will probably be better to attempt the journey down rather than sit and wait for help to arrive and run the risk of hypothermia in the meantime. Each case differs, and you will have to judge the best course of action at the time. But most victims of arm and shoulder injuries do find that they can make their own way down as long as their legs have escaped any injury in the accident. If the victim wants to walk down unaided, this is one occasion when the immobilization of the injured limb may be very helpful. Follow the usual rules: do not do anything you feel incompetent to do; be guided by the victim himself; do whatever he tells you to bring him relief from pain even if it doesn't fit in exactly with text-book drawings of what supported arms should look like.

When Might They Happen?

These fractures frequently occur as a result of a fall, if the victim puts out his hand to try to break the fall and lands on that side of his body. A slip on wet rock or grass, walking uphill or downhill, is another common cause.

What Do They Look Like?

You may be unable to tell by looking whether a fracture has occurred or not if the break is under the skin. But if you actually hear the crack of a bone as the victim falls, you can be fairly certain that a fracture has occurred, and you should proceed as though it has. It is better to over-estimate the damage rather than under-estimate it. Soon the affected area, or an area near it, will start to swell and look bruised and deformed, and the victim will be unable to move his arm, hand or fingers normally.

What Can I Do?

First, control any bleeding that might occur in the event of a compound fracture. Then proceed as follows to immobilize the limb:

Fracture of the shoulder blade or collar bone:

1. Place some sort of padding in the victim's armpit. If you have insufficient material in the first-aid kit, improvise with handkerchiefs, thick tissues or any soft material.
2. Use a triangular bandage from the kit to make a sling to hold the arm on the injured side in the most comfortable position, which is likely to be bent at the elbow.
3. When you have found the most comfortable resting position, hold the arm gently in place and secure it to the chest, using a broad bandage.

Fracture of the arm:

1. If the break is in the upper arm or forearm and has not affected the elbow, put the forearm gently across the chest, with the victim's fingers touching the opposite armpit.
2. Use padding to separate the arm from the chest.
3. Let the victim find the best position for the arm to rest in and support it there in a sling. Then secure the sling to the chest with a broad bandage over the sling.
4. If the elbow cannot be bent, the arm must be immobilized by bandaging it to the chest and trunk with the arm downwards. This will make it impractical for the victim to walk, and may thus defeat the object of immobilization. Either leave the fracture unbandaged, so that the victim can walk freely, or, if he finds it too painful, you will have to send for help.

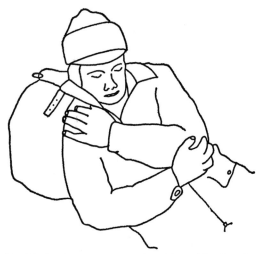

Fig. 21. Finding the most comfortable position for a fractured arm.

Fracture of the wrist and lower end of the arm:

Use padding to protect the affected area. When you have found what position is most comfortable, secure the arm in a sling, and tie a broad bandage over the sling to hold it in place, so that the arm stays bent against the chest.

Can I Give a Drink?

A small cup of water or tea or soup may help comfort the victim if he particularly requests it. Otherwise, do not give a drink.

Of the Pelvis

This serious fracture usually results from a heavy fall which may well have caused other injuries. The fracture itself may also have damaged internal organs, particularly the bladder.

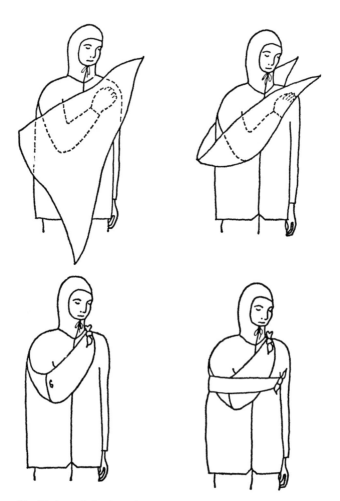

Fig. 22. Immobilization of right arm using triangular bandage and broad bandage.

When Might It Happen?

A fractured pelvis is a typical rock-climbing injury, following a heavy fall when the casualty lands on his feet.

What Does It Look Like?

It can be very difficult to identify this sort of fracture because there is often no sign at all of injury to the lower half of the body. However, there are other clues you can follow. The victim will feel pain in his hips and loins which gets worse if he moves or coughs. He may not be able to stand. If he has to pass water, serious internal injuries may be indicated by blood colouring the urine.

What Can I Do?

1. Concentrate all your efforts on getting help as soon as possible.

2. Do not move the victim. Transportation of this sort of injury is a highly specialized job, not to be undertaken by the inexperienced, who could even kill the victim.

3. Comfort and reassure the victim, and keep him moderately warm without overheating him. If the victim is lying on his back, he may be a little more comfortable if he lies either with his knees straight or slightly bent. If bent, you can support them by using a rucksack placed gently under the knees.

Can I Give a Drink?

Yes, in small sips.

Of the Thigh (Femur)

This can be a very serious fracture because it often gives rise to considerable internal bleeding which causes shock, and also because the strong muscles in this part of the leg react to the fracture by contracting and displacing the broken ends of the bone, thus causing much pain for the victim.

When Might It Happen?

It most often occurs as a result of a fall, which is a common type of accident on the hills.

What Does It Look Like?

A characteristic sign of a fractured thigh, or femur, is that one leg, the injured one, will appear shorter than the other. This is because the thigh muscles go into spasm, displacing the bone ends. When this part of the leg is broken, the foot will probably lie parallel to the ground. If the fracture is

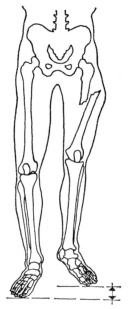

Fig. 23. Fractured femur showing shortening of injured leg.

open, or compound, and the bone pokes through the skin, there may be considerable external bleeding. Sometimes, the force of the strong muscles contracting can actually push the broken thigh bone through the skin. The victim will be in great pain.

What Can I Do?

First you must concentrate on the essentials and then if you feel confident enough to take steps to reduce the pain, there are further measures to be taken.

1. The victim is likely to be losing a lot of blood, so control the bleeding, and treat him for shock (see page 153). Reassure him and comfort him, and keep him protected from the cold.

2. You will certainly need help to get the victim off the hills, so send for assistance without delay.

3. If you are a long way from help, perhaps several hours, or even overnight, and if the victim is in great pain, you can help by doing something fairly simple called 'traction'. This is just stretching the leg to ease the tight muscles and relieve the pain that they are causing around the fracture. First, secure the victim to a stable point like a rock or tree by using a rucksack to strap him to it, as illustrated. Then take the foot of the injured leg between your hands, one at the heel and one round the toes, and pull gently towards you, stretching the injured leg out straight. This should prevent the taut muscles from displacing the bone and bring some relief from the pain.

4. Generally, it is unnecessary for you to immobilize a fracture of the thigh because the rescue party will do this before they carry the casualty down the hill. However, there is always the chance that you may have to do it one day, so it is as well to know how. Pad out the space between the injured and uninjured leg with soft material, and then tie the injured leg with triangular bandages to the uninjured one. Never tie these too tightly. The injured area may swell,

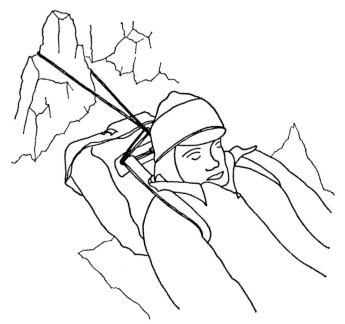

Fig. 24. Securing victim to fixed point.

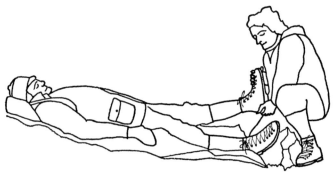

. 25. Traction of the femur.

and tight bandages could interfere with circulation. If the bone is poking through the skin in the case of a compound fracture, cover it loosely with a clean triangular bandage and pack the wound with gauze on the outside.

Can I Give a Drink?

As in most cases involving fractures, it is better to avoid giving a drink unless the victim wants one very badly, in which case give just one small cup of water, tea or soup.

Of the Lower Leg and Ankle

These fractures, which are often compound or open breaks, occur in the same instances as fractures of the femur and can be treated in much the same way, although you will not need to stretch the leg in traction because there will not be such painful muscular reaction.

When Might It Happen?

Often after a fall or a blow from a falling boulder.

What Can I Do?

1. Comfort and reassure the victim, minimize shock, protect him from the cold and send for help if this is practical and a rescue party can reach you in reasonable time.

2. If rescue is on its way, leave the immobilization of the broken bone to the team members. However, if you have no alternative but to carry out your own evacuation, then you will have to immobilize the fracture.

3. As for the thigh – pad out the hollow between the injured and uninjured legs, then secure the injured leg to the good one using triangular bandages. Tie them loosely enough to allow for the swelling which follows a fracture.

Can I Give a Drink?

Not unless particularly requested.

Of the Foot

Even if you wear the best boots available for the country in which you are walking or climbing, unfortunately they cannot protect your feet from all kinds of accident.

When Might It Happen?

A foot can be broken, or the bone crushed, by the weight of a falling boulder (especially on scree slopes) or by any considerable weight falling from above. Take comfort from the facts that at least the foot is less seriously damaged than the skull if hit in this way, and a strong boot does give you some protection.

What Does It Look Like?

You will not be able to see very much without removing the boot, if you can take it off easily. The foot will be swollen and bruised and gradually it will appear deformed when compared with the uninjured foot.

What Can I Do?

1. If the victim is unable to walk, you will have to send for help. If he attempts to get down unaided, he may put extra strain on the good foot and fall again.

2. If you cannot remove the boot easily, leave it on and give the foot extra support with padding. Then tie a broad bandage over the boot and round the ankle in the figure of eight.

3. If the boot can be taken off easily, slide it off very gently and find the injured area. If you have to carry the victim down, immobilize the foot by securing it to the uninjured foot using padding and a broad bandage.

4. If you have no choice but for the victim to walk down rather than being carried, leave the padded boot on the injured foot secured gently with a broad bandage, and find a stick for the victim to help take his weight as he hobbles down.

In all cases of simple fractures, dislocations and sprains, a cold compress can be made from bandages soaked in cold water, and this will reduce swelling and bruising.

Of the Spine

Because of the complicated and serious nature of spinal fractures and injuries, the spine is dealt with separately on page 162.

FROSTNIP AND FROSTBITE

To most people the word frostbite conjures up images of intrepid explorers conquering unbeaten peaks in the Himalayas under extreme conditions and often arriving home minus fingers and toes, which they have sacrificed to frostbite for the sake of the great challenge. But you don't have to bivouac half-way up Everest to get frostbite. Given the right circumstances frostbite (and, less seriously, frost-nip) does occur in this country. It is more easily avoidable than hypothermia, and once you understand what exactly causes it and what happens, you can take precautions to prevent it.

Hypothermia is usually caused by the combination of wind and wet, which is a very common British weather pattern, and also one which is not always predictable, so that walkers and climbers who start out in fine weather can end up as hypothermia victims simply because they were unable to foresee rapid weather changes. Frostbite is not such a random mishap. It often occurs in very cold, dry, fine conditions when the victim is inadequately protected against the cold, or when something like a very tight boot impedes the circulation of the blood which controls heat regulation. The sequence of events is, in principle, quite similar to that in hypothermia. When the body's inner vital core containing the essential parts of the body such as the heart, lungs and liver becomes chilled, it automatically robs the outer parts, including the hands and feet, of heat to keep the inner core supplied with enough warmth to continue functioning. When this happens, and the atmospheric temperature is below freezing, the outer extremities, deprived of their normal heat, literally become frozen. The tissues freeze, and ice crystals form in between the surrounding cells. The degrees of seriousness of frostbite range from the very superficial, when the cells are not irreversibly damaged, to the very extreme deep frostbite, when prolonged freezing kills the cells, makes the area very receptive to infection and eventually causes the loss of the affected part which has to be amputated. This type of deep frostbite would be very unusual in Britain, but milder forms of the condition, especially frostnip, are quite common.

Frostnip is the first sign of frostbite, and if the right action is taken at this early warning stage frostbite need never follow.

When Is It Likely to Happen?

Frostnip occurs when temperatures are below freezing, when either you are not wearing enough warm clothing or you have left parts of your body, such as your hands or face, exposed too long in the severe cold. It can also happen if you are walking in snow wearing shoes with thin soles providing poor insulation from the cold, or if you have your boots tied so tightly that you cut off circulation to the feet. Lack of sufficient food before facing extreme cold can contribute to its onset.

What Does It Look Like?

You can see frostnip developing as well as feeling it, so that you can spot the danger signals and act quickly. The victim loses feeling in the affected area, and his fingers, toes, nose or cheeks feel numb after having felt very cold. The skin in the numb area goes white and waxy-looking. As soon as this happens, you must rewarm the affected part to prevent the frostnip from becoming frostbite and penetrating deeper under the skin.

What Can I Do?

You should use the body's areas of warmth to restore heat in a gentle but rapid way.

1. If the victim's cheeks or nose are white and numb, use the palms of the hand to cover them, or breathe onto the area until the colour is restored and the warmth returned. Don't rub or chafe the skin.

2. If the hands are numbed, rewarm them either by putting one of the victim's hands under each of your armpits inside your clothing, so that your warm skin will transmit heat gently to the cold fingers, or else let him rewarm them by heat from between his thighs inside his clothing.

3. If the feet are affected, remove the victim's boots and socks and sit on the ground so that he can put both feet against the warm skin under your anorak and sweaters. Once again, don't rub or chafe the numb area. As feeling returns, the skin may sting and tingle.

4. If you take this action at an early stage, no further damage will result and all that remains to be done is to make sure that the frostnipped fingers or face are not left exposed again, or the condition will recur.

If feeling fails to return to the numb area in a short time and the white appearance of the skin does not change, you must assume that you have a case of frostbite, since the outward appearance is no different. This will mean that the freezing has affected deeper tissue. There is no first-aid treatment suitable for this condition that you can give on the hills. Rewarming must be done under finely controlled conditions by experts.

In any case of frost damage, whether minor or serious, NEVER act as follows:

1. NEVER rub or chafe numb parts to restore warmth. If the frostbite has damaged tissue under the skin, this will make the risk of infection even greater if you happen to break the skin. This action will neither melt the frozen cells nor improve circulation.

2. NEVER rub snow on the affected parts for the same reason.

3. NEVER use direct heat, such as the flame of a lighter or match or fire, or hot water, to try to restore feeling to the dead part. Rewarming must be done under supervision. In more serious cases it is better to walk down the hill with the limb still in its frozen state, even if it is a foot, than partially to reheat it before the journey down, only to let it cool again.

HEAD INJURIES

Emergency Action Quick Reference

1. Check immediately that the victim is still breathing and that his heart is beating. If deeply unconscious, suffocation may follow rapidly if the tongue causes airway blockage. Clear airway without delay and start artificial resuscitation (see page 58).

2. Control external bleeding (see page 68) but don't exert direct pressure over any broken skull bones.

3. If possible keep an accurate written record of any changes in the condition of an unconscious victim.

4. Get help as a matter of urgency.

Head injuries on the hills are usually caused by falls from crags or down steep slopes, and by rocks and stones dislodged from above. The injuries can vary from very simple cuts to concussion and brain damage. Ten years ago, it was unusual to see climbers wearing protective helmets, but the wisdom of wearing them has now become generally accepted, to the extent that climbers may be considered badly equipped without them. Helmets have helped to reduce the numbers of head injuries. However, many climbers choose not to wear them, and they are not considered to be necessary for hill-walking. So head injuries continue to occur.

In any case of head injury, you should suspect concussion. This is a sort of brain-shaking, and is indicated by unconsciousness, even if only for a moment. It can be caused by a fall in which the victim lands very heavily on both feet and jolts the rest of his body, as well as by direct impact to the head. Concussion can be accompanied by stoppage of the heart and of breathing. A further complication of a direct blow on the head could be a fracture of the skull, which may damage blood vessels. Any consequent bleeding beneath the skull can cause compression of the brain, because the swelling and bleeding is confined within the skull. This can lead to irreparable brain damage.

What Should I Notice?

You can never be certain of the extent of the damage after the head has been injured. External bleeding will be obvious if you look and feel for any damp patches of blood obscured by hair, but concussion and compression may not be.

In cases of concussion the victim loses consciousness, perhaps only for a moment; breathing will be shallow and the face looks pale. His skin will feel clammy and cold if you touch it, and his pulse is rapid and weak. If he comes round, he may vomit, and will probably have no recollection of the accident which caused the injury or the events leading up to it.

However, if the more serious injury of brain compression is occurring, that is, if a broken skull bone or escaping blood are putting pressure on the brain, the victim breathes noisily and his face looks flushed and hot. His pulse becomes slow and the pupils of his eyes look unequal in size, or very enlarged, and unresponsive to light. You can carry out a

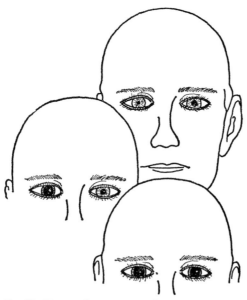

Fig. 26. Abnormal appearance of eye pupils indicating serious head injury.

quick test to ascertain this by shining a light, like a torch, into the eyes and seeing if the pupils respond. In addition to these irregular eye responses, you may also notice weakness or paralysis down one side of the body.

What Can I Do?

1. Always check that the victim is breathing and that his heart is beating. In addition to the danger of brain damage, deep unconsciousness may cause an airway blockage because the tongue falls backwards blocking the

throat, and in this state the victim will be unable to make any automatic response to help himself to start breathing again. In fact, most fatalities following head injuries are caused by this type of suffocation, so be prepared to start artificial resuscitation immediately (see page 54).

2. It may be difficult to control any external bleeding if the fracture has caused broken bones to protrude through the skin, but whatever you do avoid putting on the bones themselves any pressure which could drive them back into the skull. As with all compound fractures, cut a hole in the dressing and let the broken bones poke through.

3. Don't be tempted to dismiss a head injury as very slight – the accident may have caused bleeding inside the skull and the escaping blood eventually presses on the brain. Collapse could occur at any time, even when you think the victim is recovering.

4. If the victim is unconscious, keep an accurate record (written down if at all possible) of any changes you notice in his condition. It may be easier for a doctor to assess the extent of serious brain damage if he has a complete picture of the patient's progress or deterioration in the first few minutes, or hours, after the accident. Check any changes which occur to the pupils of the eyes, for example their size and response to light, and with each entry on the record note the time. Check also to see if there is any discharge of blood or fluid from the ears which may indicate very serious head injury. If you notice this, record it, with the time, and do no more than cover the ear with a dressing.

5. Send for help urgently. Whether the victim is conscious or not, he will require assistance down the hill, and in any event further complications may arise. In a very remote and dangerous situation, where the wait for assistance could bring risks of exposure for instance, a conscious victim will have to be helped to safety, but first allow as much recovery time as possible – there is a danger of further collapse if brain compression has occurred. Moving an unconscious victim without expert assistance is extremely dangerous because the full extent of injury will be unknown and any

rough handling on the journey down could paralyse or kill. Such moving should only be attempted to avoid death from other factors.

Can I Give a Drink?

No. Don't give a drink even if the victim becomes fully conscious and alert.

HEART ATTACK

Emergency Action Quick Reference

1. In case of unconscious collapse, check immediately to see if heart or breathing have failed.
2. Start artificial resuscitation (see page 54) at once, if necessary, using cardiac compression and mouth-to-mouth assisted breathing.
3. Continue resuscitation and send for help urgently.
4. In the case of conscious victim, make him comfortable, loosen any tight clothing and send for help urgently.

Heart attack, or coronary thrombosis, is the commonest of the more serious illnesses occurring on the hills and it is something about which you can do very little to help once it has happened. A fair number of these cases end in almost immediate death. Every year the hills of Britain claim an increasing toll of such victims, probably for the simple reason that proportionately more people of all age groups are discovering the challenges of walking and climbing, and thus a correspondingly larger number of them come to grief when facing the physical strain that their hill exploits impose. However, some attacks are less serious than others, and it is very well worthwhile knowing just what limited help you can give, even if it should ultimately fail.

What Happens When a Victim Suffers a Heart Attack?

Usually, an essential vessel carrying blood to the heart becomes blocked, often by a blood clot, thus preventing the necessary supply of blood from reaching the heart muscle. Those most at risk are middle-aged people who are already suffering from a disease which has caused their blood vessels to become narrower than they should be. However, attacks can strike even those in the early thirties. Strenuous exercise, especially in the unfit, demands more oxygen, and to provide this the heart increases the rate of blood circulation. If this suddenly increased volume of blood is trying to force its way through abnormally narrow channels, the blockage can occur which gives rise to the heart attack.

Warnings may be felt in the form of chest pains, known as angina. If the victim is lucky enough to have early warning, he must stop and rest immediately or worse may follow. Some people live with angina for years and know what they must do when they feel these danger signs. It can be very difficult even for experts to distinguish between angina and a mild heart attack, but it really isn't necessary for the first-aider to know any more than that any heart pain is either instantly or potentially very serious and cannot be taken lightly.

What Will I Notice?

Apart from chest pains, the victim of a heart attack or angina will feel a constricting of the chest. The pain may also affect his arms and neck. Breathing will be difficult and you may see a bluish tinge around the lips. The victim may complain of pain or think that he has indigestion, and the attack may come during the strenuous exercise or just after it – in fact it is more common for the victim to start the attack during descent, when the going is easier, rather than during the climb uphill. If these symptoms are followed rapidly by collapse, act quickly.

What Can I Do?

1. Check that the casualty is breathing and that his heart is beating. If either have failed, start artificial resuscitation without delay (see page 54). Be prepared for vomiting, and if this occurs turn him quickly on his side to prevent choking.

2. Continue assisted breathing and cardiac massage for as long as necessary, and send for help urgently.

If the victim is still conscious and has not collapsed:

1. Help him to sit down on the ground in the most comfortable position for him, and, if there is nothing like a wall or a rock for him to lean against, make a support for his

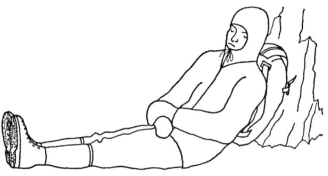

Fig. 27. Comfortable position for conscious heart-attack victim.

back with rucksacks and spare clothing. If he prefers to rest at a lower angle, help him find the most comfortable position, lying down but with his head slightly raised.

2. Check that he is not wearing any tight clothing. If he is, loosen it.

3. Talk to him calmly and quietly. If he is able to reply, try to find out whether he has ever had similar pains, and, if he knows that he has angina, whether he is carrying a supply of drugs with him to help ease the pain. Reassure

him, and don't let him feel anxious about anything because this could make his condition worse.

4. Even if he recovers, don't suggest continuing the walk. Send for help, as he should be carried down.

5. Keep a constant check on him in case the first pains are followed by a heart attack, and be ready to start artificial resuscitation in case he becomes unconscious at any stage.

Can I Give a Drink?

If the victim is fully conscious and not likely to choke, a drink may be given in small sips.

If you are walking with a middle-aged person whom you know to have a history of heart trouble, avoid a long tiring walk at high levels in isolated country far removed from help. Make sure that the person is carrying any necessary drugs in a place that you can find easily and that he understands that, while it is his own personal decision to take what risks may be involved for him in hill-walking, his enjoyment should not be at the expense of putting anybody else's life at risk should he need rescuing from a remote place in bad conditions.

HEATSTROKE

In the past, heatstroke has not been a common hazard in our normally temperate climate, but the period of unusually hot weather in the summer of 1976 caused quite large numbers of people to collapse from the effects of excessive heat. Health authorities estimated that a three-week heat wave in June 1976 contributed to the deaths of 3,000 people who would not otherwise have died at that time. In the same month, many walkers on the mountains of Britain collapsed in varying stages of exhaustion and dehydration.

Experts say that high temperatures in summer are not simply freak conditions, and predict that they may follow a regular pattern for the next few years. With temperatures as high as 32°C in the shade, prolonged physical exertion in direct sunlight can easily result in excessive loss of body fluid through perspiration, which will cause heatstroke if not corrected.

When we exert energy in heat, we sweat, and if we overheat too much, we sweat too much and lose fluid and salt. The first stage of heatstroke is often cramp, due to the salt deficiency.

The next stage may be rather more dramatic: Sometimes the victim of excessive heat starts feeling weary, and then turns quite pale and eventually faints, or even vomits. If you touch him, he feels clammy and breathes quickly.

If the heat is very excessive, or if there is high humidity as well, the dangerous stage of heatstroke can follow. High humidity can prevent the evaporation of sweat and accelerate the eventual breakdown of the body's devices for regulating its temperature. The result can be sudden fever, followed by unconsciousness and death.

First aid can be very effective at all stages. The normal practice of keeping the victim warm is reversed, and the first-aider instead must use all his ingenuity in keeping the victim cool. If the first sign of heatstroke is cramp, act as follows:

1. If you have any salt, add about half a teaspoon to a pint of water and give it to the victim to drink. This should make him feel better very rapidly, because it is directly replacing the salt and fluid which the body has just lost.

2. To relieve the pain caused by the cramp, help the victim to stretch the affected leg muscles as described on pages 86–8. If the cramp eases and the victim recovers, it should be quite safe for you to go slowly down the hill with him. Don't try to complete your planned walk for the day, because heatstroke can easily recur. If the cramp doesn't stop and the victim continues to feel ill, call for help and

wait with him in the shade, giving him plenty to drink and glucose in the form of sweets or fruit squash, which will provide fluid and glucose together.

If the heat makes the victim faint, the first aid is similar:

1. Let the victim recover in the position in which he has collapsed before trying to move him, if this is practical and he is not in a dangerous place. Keep the direct sun off him and help him to cool down by removing unnecessary clothing – he may be suffering because he is wearing unsuitably warm clothes.

2. When he is fully conscious, give him a drink of water with a little salt in it, but be sparing with the salt in case it makes him feel sick. Be very careful when giving a drink that the victim doesn't choke and don't let him gulp it down too fast; instead give it in small sips.

3. Allow plenty of time resting in the cool before attempting to help the victim down. If you are in any doubt at all about whether or not the casualty is fit enough to walk down, then call for help, in case the heatstroke recurs more seriously.

If the victim is showing all these signs of the ill effects of the heat, don't waste time. Call for help immediately, while keeping him as cool and quiet as possible. You could wipe his face with dressings and bandages out of the first-aid kit dipped in cold water to make him feel more comfortable. Reassure him, and do not let him get anxious.

Heatstroke is easily avoidable, and, if the hot summer is to become a part of our climate, we shall all have to learn how to behave in extreme heat to prevent illness. Some of the most fundamental lessons can be learnt from the people of traditionally warm countries. For instance, it would be very unusual to see a Southern European toiling up a steep hill in the direct midday sun wearing thick clothes and carrying a heavy pack. If it is very hot, and humid as well, avoid walking on the hills at all until a cooler part of the day. With the long light summer evenings this is not an impractical suggestion. If you think the weather may be very warm, carry salt tablets with you and use them as directed. These can be bought at any chemist and kept as an additional summer item in the first-aid kit. Drink plenty of water, do not burden yourself with a heavy pack, and wear light clothing which will absorb the sweat. If you still want to walk in very hot weather, be sensible and give in at the first sign of exhaustion. You won't enjoy the walk in conditions like this anyway. If you are walking on a set route as part of some sort of endurance test or award scheme, you must be ready to admit defeat once the extreme heat really fatigues you, just as you should admit defeat in any bad conditions. If you don't, you could cause a lot of people to go to considerable expense and trouble on your behalf.

HYPOTHERMIA

Conditions and Symptoms

1. Cold, wet, windy weather.
2. Physical exhaustion, hunger and anxiety.
3. Uncharacteristic actions or speech (speech may also be slurred).
4. Lethargy, cramp, stumbling and fits of violent shivering.

NB: Not all of these symptoms are necessarily present together.

Emergency Action Quick Reference

1. Make the victim STOP.
2. Insulate him from the cold, using spare clothing, or put him inside a plastic exposure bag with a fit person.
3. Erect a tent or makeshift shelter round him.
4. Give him warm sweet drinks, or food such as chocolate containing glucose.

5. Send for help urgently, and be ready at any time to give artificial resuscitation (see page 54).

Over the last few years, 'hypothermia' has become one of the most fashionable words in the world of outdoor activities, and yet for all the publicity it is still one of the least understood and most dangerous risks in mountain pursuits. Given the right conditions, which are frequent in Britain, it can affect entire parties. Young people especially have been unexpectedly caught by this extraordinarily swift death.

Hypothermia is one of the most important conditions for the first-aider to understand because first aid can be the only aid. If it fails, it may be too late for experienced help to do much, and a mistake in the early stages is often irreversible, because time is so limited. Hypothermia is not a condition exclusive to areas like the Alps or Himalayas, the Polar regions or mountains of any particular height. It can, and does, occur in most parts of Britain during *every month of the year* if certain weather conditions prevail. The killing factor is the insidious, creeping nature of the condition which affects the mind and body at the same time, so that, unless you know just what the warning signs are, hypothermia can overtake a whole group of people in rapid succession. If hypothermia and its dangers were understood more widely, the death toll from incidents on British mountains could be cut drastically.

It is therefore essential to know just what hypothermia is; when it is likely to occur; what happens when it does, and what danger signs to look for; and what to do next before it is too late . . . and what not to do.

What Is It?

To understand hypothermia, it is necessary to understand how the body manages to heat itself normally. You can divide the body roughly into two sections. At the centre is the core, which contains the vital organs including the heart, lungs, liver and brain. This core is kept at a constant temperature by certain automatic heat regulators. The rest of the body forms a shell of the surface layers around the core, the lower part of the belly, arms and legs. The two sections interact constantly to maintain core heat but this regulation of heat cannot work efficiently if external cold, like wind and rain together, penetrate the protective outer shell. It is when this chilling reaches the core that we say the victim has hypothermia, and the heat essential to the core escapes into the shell. This usually occurs when the core temperature drops below 35°C (95°F). At this stage, the automatic heating regulation system breaks down, and active artificial measures to rewarm the central core have to be taken rapidly to prevent death. However, many complicated factors are involved in rewarming, and it can be fatal to do it in the wrong way. For example, a first-aider might decide that a generous swig of brandy, in the best Alpine tradition, was all that was needed. The tot of alcohol will effectively cause blood vessels in the cooler outer shell of the body to send a sudden flow of the cooler blood to the already rapidly cooling core, resulting in an even greater heat loss. So you see that unless you understand what your first aid is actually doing, it could be fatal.

What Sort of Weather Conditions Can Cause It?

Although any one of the following factors can cause hypothermia, it is normally the result of a combination of several. All are familiar conditions in Britain. They are cold, wind and wetness, which, if combined with fatigue, injury, illness, unfitness, inadequate clothing or lack of food, can rapidly cause death. Here is a typical story:

Two young men take a weekend off from their home town and head for the mountains, where they have both enjoyed camping and walking during the summer. It is early spring, and they know the area fairly well. They set off from the warm valley after a lie-in and brew-up about

11 a.m. in bright sunshine. They have planned a route for a day's walk and they have a map, but there's nobody around, so they don't tell anyone where they are going, or leave a note on their tent or motor-bike. They haven't got much cash to spare, so, although they both are wearing good boots, they wear the clothes they usually wear out of doors – jeans, a sweater and a showerproof anorak each. By lunchtime, they have climbed to about 1,500 feet, but it has started to cloud over and by 2 p.m. it is pouring with rain. They shelter, but their jeans are wet and the anoraks cannot keep the wet out for very long. They walk on, because the rain doesn't stop, then the wind gets up as well, and before long they start to feel cold. They've eaten the food they had with them hours ago, and they start to feel a little anxious about finishing the route, but they can't take a short cut down very easily because they don't recognize where they are now that low cloud has blotted out the surrounding hills, and they haven't got a compass. So they keep on going in the direction that they think they should be heading. One suddenly starts acting the fool, and staggering and lurching as if he is drunk. The other asks him what sort of game he thinks he's playing, and a row develops because the first says he feels cold and wants to have a rest. The other is very anxious by now because it won't be light for very much longer, but he finds that he's not too quick at making decisions and feels a little hazy himself. He eventually decides that the best thing to do is to carry on regardless, so he tells his companion to pull himself together and keep walking. They stagger on shivering until both collapse, and their bodies are not found for two days because nobody knew they were missing, or where to start looking.

This tale is no stretch of the imagination. It is characteristic of deaths which happen every year from Dartmoor to Skye. The weather combinations most likely to cause hypothermia occur more frequently in Britain than elsewhere in Europe, and within Britain are the two wettest European mountain areas, the Scafell Cirque and the Snowdon Basin. Most of the rain is accompanied by a brisk prevailing south-west wind. The wind alone is a major hazard. Most of us associate the presence of freezing rain, sleet or snow with severe conditions, but few people realize that a 25 m.p.h. wind in a temperature of 20°F is equivalent to a temperature of −15°F.

Wind Chill Chart

ESTIMATED WIND SPEED IN M.P.H.	ACTUAL THERMOMETER READING (°F)											
	50	40	30	20	10	0	-10	-20	-30	-40	-50	-60
	EQUIVALENT TEMPERATURE (°F)											
calm	50	40	30	20	10	0	-10	-20	-30	-40	-50	-60
5	48	37	27	16	6	-5	-15	-26	-36	-47	-57	-68
10	40	28	16	4	-9	-21	-33	-46	-58	-70	-83	-95
15	36	22	9	-5	-18	-36	-45	-58	-72	-85	-99	-112
20	32	18	4	-10	-25	-39	-53	-67	-82	-96	-110	-124
25	30	16	0	-15	-29	-44	-59	-74	-88	-104	-118	-133
30	28	13	-2	-18	-33	-48	-63	-79	-94	-109	-125	-140
35	27	11	-4	-20	-35	-49	-67	-82	-98	-113	-129	-145
40	26	10	-6	-21	-37	-53	-69	-85	-100	-116	-132	-148

(wind speeds greater than 40 m.p.h. have little additional effect)	LITTLE DANGER (for properly clothed person)	Increasing DANGER	GREAT DANGER
		Danger from freezing of exposed flesh	

How Can I Recognize It?

Hypothermia can be so difficult to recognize that by the time you are aware that something is wrong it may be too late. For this reason, you must be extremely observant and vigilant in noticing anything amiss in bad weather conditions, not just to protect yourself but to help those people who may not understand the dangers.

The first important factor is weather, as already described. If any combination of wet, cold, wind or exhaustion is present, start being wary. Notice also what your companions are wearing, and if you see wet jeans or a torn kagoule or an uncovered head, be even more watchful. (Perhaps you should have noticed these clothing deficiencies before you started out and mentioned them, but it is too late now, even if better gear was available.) Did you have breakfast together before you set out, and if so what sort of meal was it? What kind of food are your friends carrying, and have they eaten anything since they started out? Being aware of these small details may help you to identify possible victims, but there are more definite signs which mean that trouble has already arrived.

1. The onset of hypothermia can cause changes in the normal pattern of behaviour, and one of the first symptoms is often rather odd or uncharacteristic actions or speech. It helps if you know the victim well enough to be able to assess any change in mood, but the sort of thing you should notice is a sudden display of temper or aggression in normally quiet people, or a sudden careless action in a normally careful person.

2. At the same time, the victim often complains of cold, tiredness and cramp, but if the hypothermia is already well advanced the cold may have affected his brain: he will become increasingly confused or lethargic and may be unable to say what is wrong. In this state, he will find it very difficult to understand or answer simple questions or directions, and yet if you suggest any sort of help your concern may well be met with aggression. The victim might even try to fight you off in your attempt to stop him walking.

3. He may also stagger and stumble in a typically drunken manner. His speech may be slurred and his vision may also be affected.

4. The victim may be having fits of violent shivering. If you see any of these signs, or a combination of several, the condition is already very far advanced and you will have to act very quickly to prevent collapse and death.

If any of these signs are apparent in one person, they could soon show in other members of the party. Some people are more susceptible to hypothermia than others (for example, anyone taking certain types of drugs including tranquillizers could find it harder to deal with low temperatures) and, although the dangerous weather conditions affect the weakest first, next in line come the stronger. Before long even the hardiest person in the party could be fighting for his life against the fatal combination of wet, wind and exhaustion.

What Can I Do?

You can save life by doing nothing more difficult than using common sense and ingenuity. The first part of your life-saving action should have been the careful observation just described. If you do this soon enough, and then carry out the second part of the first aid, there is every chance that you will all survive. This is what you must do next:

1. STOP, wherever you are, even if there is no shelter. Naturally, if you can see shelter very near, make for it, but don't continue to walk on in the hope of finding shelter.

2. Choose the fittest people to go for help immediately (see page 43).

3. If you are carrying camping gear, much of your equipment can be put to good use. Insulate the victim from the cold ground with spare clothing or a groundsheet to prevent further heat loss, cover him with all available spare sweaters, then put him inside a plastic exposure bag, if possible together with a fit person.

4. Meanwhile, if there are enough of you, put up a tent if you have one. If you have, you probably have sleeping-bags as well, so put a sleeping-bag inside the tent, and let one of the fittest members of the group strip to his underclothes and get in the bag, to warm it in readiness for the victim.

5. When you have done that, carry the victim with his head at a downwards angle to the tent, strip wet clothing off him, and put him in the sleeping-bag with the fit person, so that his warmth can help warm the victim. No doubt it will be a tight squeeze to fit two people in the bag, but huddle as close as possible to the victim, and, while you must not rub his skin, if the bag is large enough you could help to warm his hands and feet by putting them under your arm-pits, and between your thighs just below the groin.

6. If you have a tent and a sleeping-bag, with any luck you will have some sort of equipment on which to cook or make hot drinks, unless you are carrying Thermos flasks. Brew up as soon as you can, inside the tent if possible to warm it up, although this is rather a dangerous practice under normal circumstances. If the victim is conscious and there is no danger of his choking, give him warm, sweet drinks and energy-producing foods such as chocolate, nuts, raisins, Kendal Mintcake or any sugary snacks you may have, or even the condensed milk in a tube which some campers carry.

7. Although you must concentrate all your efforts for the time being on the victim, at the same time keep a watchful eye on everybody in the party including yourself to make sure that you are not showing similar symptoms. Keep as warm as possible, wear all spare clothing available and even use your empty rucksack to insulate your legs and feet.

8. Even if the victim seems to be recovering, stay put if possible and wait for help to arrive. It is not practical to make general and definite rules to cover every single case of hypothermia, but remember that if you notice the danger signs in time and act quickly and the victim seems to be recovering, not much harm will come to you by staying put where you are until help arrives. As usual, the difficulty lies in the remotest parts of Scotland, where help may be days away, and it could be dangerous to wait. If you have to move, wait as long as you can for the victim to recover before attempting any sort of evacuation. Be prepared for the hypothermia to come again – frequent stops may be necessary. The choice is not an easy one, and the alternatives equally grim. You could either wait for a partial recovery and then try to reach safety at the risk of killing the victim on the way; or you could stay put hoping that dogs and rescuers will find you before your food and fuel run out. If you have adequate equipment, on balance it would be wiser to stay put, but you may prefer to take a chance on meeting the rescuers half-way.

What Can I Do without Tent, Extra Clothing or Food?

1. STOP. If you can reach a natural shelter within yards, use it, otherwise stop where you are.

2. Lay the victim down, after putting some sort of insulation under his body between him and the ground. Try to put up a makeshift shelter using rocks, branches, rucksacks or even hardpacked snow to form a wall which will protect the victim from driving rain, snow or cold wind.

3. Send the fittest members of the party for help, if you have not done so already, while the remaining people in the group huddle together as closely as possible, with one lying each side of the victim hugging him to try and transfer warmth to him from their bodies. Breathe out warm air over his face, and put his hands under someone else's clothing. If you have an exposure bag, and you should have one as part of basic equipment, get inside it with the victim in much the same way as a sleeping-bag.

4. Give the conscious victim any sort of easily digestible sweet food that you have, like chocolate, sweets and any warm sweet drinks that you may be carrying in flasks.

5. If you are out on a day's walk and so not too far away from help, stay where you are until help arrives, doing everything you can to keep the victim warm, comfortable and relaxed. In cases of hypothermia there is a serious danger of anxiety, low morale or even desperation, which can all weaken the will to survive. It is most important to keep morale as high as possible by remaining cheerful and confident.

Much research has been done recently into the best ways of caring for hypothermia victims, and chances of survival have improved a great deal in the last ten years. Sophisticated equipment and treatment techniques are now being used by rescue teams. Some have facilities at their bases for re-heating victims in warm baths at controlled temperatures. Rescue teams in the Lake District are pioneering the use of a portable reviving device which can be used on the hill, as the victim is actually being rescued, to breathe warm air into his lungs. With this sort of equipment to hand, it is most important to get expert help as soon as possible.

What NOT To Do

1. Don't give alcohol to a victim of hypothermia. It may cause a sudden rush of cold blood back to the heart from the outer surface to the inner core, and this could be fatal.

2. Don't try to rub the victim's skin in an attempt to warm him. This could once again cause a fatal rush of cool blood to the heart, or it could cause damage to underlying tissues, especially if there is also a risk of frostbite to the hands and feet. Don't rub snow on affected parts – this is another dangerous old wives' tale for treating victims of the cold, and it can make things worse.

3. Don't place a hot-water bottle against the skin of the victim. This, yet again, could cause a fatal rush of cold blood to the heart. Reheating must be done under careful medical supervision.

4. If you have done all the right things and are waiting for help to arrive, don't be tempted or persuaded to make the victim walk down himself. The condition could easily worsen or recur.

5. Never underestimate the seriousness of hypothermia. By the time you notice its presence it may already be too late, and your first aid must be rapid and correct. Hypothermia need not happen, should not happen, and may happen less if you pass the message on, and always take heed of the following:

How Can I Prevent It?

1. Before you set out, check the local weather forecast. If it predicts severe conditions or an all-day downpour, either change your route to a low-level walk or stay at home.

2. Eat a nourishing breakfast to give you plenty of energy

and carry a supply of energy-producing foods with glucose, such as chocolate, sweet drinks, raisins, nuts or Mintcake.

3. Wear sufficient clothing, and carry spare clothing. It is better to insulate the body with several layers of thinner woollen clothing than one thick layer which could easily become wet and soggy in rain. Cover your clothing with a waterproof anorak or kagoule, and over-trousers if possible. Wear two pairs of socks inside your boots and protect your head to prevent heat loss with a woollen hat or hood.

4. Carry an exposure bag as a top-priority item in your rucksack even if you are only on a day's outing.

5. Start out as early as you can in winter, to give yourself as much daylight as possible. Always tell somebody where you are going and what time you expect to be back, and leave a note pinned to your car or tent in a prominent place.

6. Never go without map and compass, and before you start, work out several quick escape routes that you could take back to safety if somebody became ill.

7. If you are venturing into wild, remote country, especially in winter, make yourself familiar with the basic skills of survival, including how to dig a snow hole.

INSECT STINGS AND BITES

Of all the winged insects buzzing over the hills of Britain, by far the most menacing are wasps and bees. In very rare cases wasp and bee stings can kill, and even if the victim does not suffer this extreme reaction, a sting is still painful and unpleasant.

What Happens When a Victim Is Stung?

Bees, wasps and hornets inject venom which, like adder venom, interferes with the clotting of the blood. Under normal circumstances, they are harmless to man, although painful. However, some people are very sensitive to these stings and can rapidly become very ill. Many of them will have already discovered their allergy and know of the dangers; often they will have been de-sensitized by drugs, or they will carry with them some kind of antidote so that if stung on the hills they can treat themselves until help arrives. In normal cases of wasp and bee stings, first aid is very simple:

What Can I Do?

1. In the case of wasps, the sting is not left behind. In time the pain eases, and the sting causes no further ill effects. If you are camping and carrying foodstuffs, you may possibly have some vinegar: this will relieve the stinging pain.

2. Bees often leave the sting behind in the skin. If you can see it, don't try to pull it out with your fingers because you may only succeed in pushing it further in, injecting more of the venom into the victim. Instead, if you have a needle or pin, sterilize it in the flame of a lighter or match and very gently ease the sting out. Don't squeeze it. If you have no suitable cream to ease the pain and if the sting still hurts when you return from the hills, try to find a little bicarbonate of soda and apply it to the sting.

A sting is normally unpleasant, but not dangerous. However, three dangers may arise after a wasp or bee sting. The first occurs when a person with a specific allergy to these stings is affected; the second if a sting is sited on a blood vessel; the third when a bee or wasp stings inside the mouth or at the back of the throat. Stings inside the mouth are extremely dangerous because if they swell sufficiently they can block the airway and the victim dies by choking.

When Can These Dangers Arise?

All such stings occur most frequently because the victim panics with fright when he sees the insect and perhaps takes a swipe at it; the insect feels under attack and stings.

Stings in the mouth and throat are rare but can happen if the victim attacks the insect with his mouth open, or when a wasp or bee is hidden in a sandwich or drink, and is swallowed, often by a child, without being noticed.

What Happens to the Victim?

If he has an allergy to stings, or if the sting hits a blood vessel, the first signs may be very similar to severe shock, followed by collapse and difficulty in breathing.

What Can I Do?

1. If the victim's heart or breathing fail, start artificial resuscitation immediately (see page 54). In cases of such extreme reaction, there is very little else you can do beyond this until help arrives.

2. If the victim is still conscious, ask him whether he knows of any allergy he may have, and if so whether he is carrying some sort of antidote to reverse the effects of the sting.

3. While the victim remains conscious, keep him completely rested and send for help urgently, with instructions to tell the rescue team precisely what has happened so that the necessary drugs may be given as soon as possible.

What Can I Do if the Victim is Stung in the Mouth or Throat?

1. Possibly the only practical way of saving a life in these circumstances, miles away from help, on the hills, could also kill the victim if done incorrectly. If the airway is completely blocked by the swollen, stung area, and the victim is choking to death, the only solution is to make an incision in his windpipe, or trachea, to make an alternative airway. However, it would be easy for an inexperienced person to cut the victim's throat. If you have no first-aid training at all, the risk of getting this life-saving technique

right first time is so enormous that it would be better to forget do-it-yourself surgery altogether and concentrate instead on getting help as soon as you can. It is a chance in ten million that you will ever need to use this technique, but if your first aid seems incomplete without learning more about it, you should attend a first-aid course.

2. Instead, as soon as the sting occurs, try to control the swelling by making the victim take mouthfuls of cold water, which he should hold in his mouth or throat before swallowing. Try also holding a cold water-soaked compress against the neck as near the swelling as you can to slow down the effects of the sting, and give yourself more time to get the casualty to safety.

3. Although you may realize the danger he is in, don't let the victim panic. Keep him reassured and quiet while he can still breathe without difficulty in case he chokes with fright.

4. If shock eventually causes heart or breathing failure, be ready to start artificial resuscitation.

Insect bites are relatively harmless compared with stings and do not pose any first-aid emergencies, although they can be of major nuisance value. There are many different types of insect on the hills of these islands. Some are capable of injecting venom into human beings, in much the same way as the adder does, while others suck human blood, particularly in the early evening, when they search for a victim for their blood meal of the day.

This hungry interest in human hosts makes insects follow the crowds, and consequently they do not normally frequent the hills in huge numbers because there are insufficient people and animals for their needs. However, those that are around will have no difficulty in smelling you out, especially if you stop to eat in the open. It is well worthwhile to know just what is buzzing around, because, while most people don't suffer unduly as the result of insect bites, others are extremely sensitive to them and may react adversely.

Mosquitoes, or gnats, usually bite humans in the evenings,

and there are two species with very severe bites which live in the rot holes of sycamores, elms and beeches. Midges bite when the wind drops, especially on the west coasts of Ireland and Scotland when the sudden calm brings them in swarms from the marshes, particularly in conditions of high humidity. Ants give tiny doses of formic acid which cause little blisters and burns, followed by irritation. Horseflies can suck blood for up to three minutes without being noticed if the victim does not feel the puncture of their fangs. They attack most commonly in hot, heavy summer weather, in damp windless conditions. Storm flies and fleas are not hill insects, but the harvester, a small red mite, is a formidable enemy in late summer if you stop and picnic on grassland, particularly in areas of chalk like the Downs of the South of England. These pests burrow into the skin and stay as unwelcome guests for about three days afterwards, causing itchy rashes a little like chickenpox. In areas where there are sheep, a human can be bitten by the tick, which normally attacks sheep. If this happens, don't try to pull the tick out of the victim's skin, where it will lie half buried. If you pull it, you simply detach its body from its mouth. Instead, wait until you reach a supply of petrol or surgical spirit and dab a tiny drop of either on the tick. This remedy will also speed up the departure of harvesters.

Reaction to bites is normally delayed by several hours, by which time the victim will probably have returned home from the walk or climb. However, very sensitive victims may suffer a rapid reaction from insects such as the horsefly and, though they are not in any danger, it may be very uncomfortable on a long day's outing. Unless you have with you a tube of cream to soothe insect bites, there is very little you can do except prevent the victim from being tempted to scratch in case this breaks the skin near the bite. If the area around it is very swollen, immerse it in cold water: this will control the swelling and relieve the itching for a while.

LIGHTNING

Emergency Action Quick Reference

1. If a victim is struck by lightning, check immediately that he is still breathing and his heart is beating. If not, begin artificial resuscitation at once (see page 54).

2. If victim is stunned, or starts to recover, treat as for shock (see page 153). The same treatment is appropriate if the victim is badly burnt.

3. Move out of danger, away from exposed ridges, and overhangs or caves situated directly under a peak.

4. Go for help, avoiding exposed ridges as you walk.

Veterans of Alpine climbing often tell of the literally hair-raising thunderstorms so common in that area, where the electrical currents in the air make metal objects hum and turn blue, and human hair stand on end. Fortunately our hills are not subject to this sort of storm, and most of us regard the possibility of being struck by lightning as extremely remote, with the same degree of fatalism as we might accept the risk of being run over by a bus. However, lightning strikes on hill-users continue to occur from time to time. The complete unpredictability of the point where a strike will happen may suggest to many that there is little use in taking steps to avoid it, but lightning often follows a characteristic pattern, and if this is understood the risks can be reduced.

Walkers and climbers are particularly at risk from lightning because they are often in, or move to, the wrong place at the wrong time; for example, sheltering under rock overhangs and boulders can make you into a convenient spark plug gap for the current; and standing on exposed ridges means there will be nothing taller near by for the lightning to hit first. For this reason being on an exposed hillside in a storm is much more dangerous than being in a car, or a building, or a city street where tall buildings may conduct the lightning to earth harmlessly. Walkers and climbers face a higher risk of being hit by lightning.

When Is Lightning Most Likely to Strike a Victim?

Lightning over the hills tends to strike the peaks and mountain tops, and any other natural projections near by, so that a person standing on top of a mountain or hill, making himself the tallest object in sight, is in danger of being struck. People often make the mistake of thinking that it is safer to shelter just under the peak, within its overhangs or caves, but these places often receive earth currents which have bounced off the peak, so lightning is quite likely to strike here. It is also dangerous to stand upright on any ridge or exposed flat ground during a storm. Walkers have been struck in such places because they thought that it would be better to keep moving.

What Happens When a Victim Is Struck?

Not all lightning kills outright. Sometimes the victim may not be directly hit but may be affected by being in the path of an earth current as it spreads out from the source of the strike. When lightning strikes, it can make the muscles contract with the shock of the current: this may prevent the victim from being able to breathe, and it may also cause his heart to stop beating. He can be knocked off his feet, and if he is near an edge at the time he could be thrown over it. In addition to the dangers of the muscular contraction, the victim may also suffer very severe burns, which, like many electrically caused burns, may prove far more serious than they look because they extend deeply under the skin.

What Can I Do?

Assuming that you are with the victim when he is struck, in order to help him you may have to put yourself at risk if the lightning continues. If the victim has been directly hit, there will be no time to look for a safer place to move him, and unless the strike has thrown him into a difficult or dangerous place, you will have to help him on the spot.

1. Check immediately that the victim is breathing and that his heart is beating. If not, apply artificial resuscitation techniques of assisted breathing (see pages 59–61) and start cardiac massage (see pages 62–3).

2. If the victim starts to recover, treat him as for shock (see page 153). This will help to lessen the dangerous effects of the strike as well as any serious burns that the victim may have.

3. If you decide to move the victim to shelter, avoid any overhang or cave situated just under a peak in case it receives earth currents from the main source as it hits the peak above; lightning *can* strike twice in the same place. Also avoid lone trees standing apart on a ridge. Instead, the safest place to be during a storm on the hills is on an open scree slope about six metres from the summit, sitting with your knees up and your hands in your lap.

4. If the victim is only stunned by the strike, get to him as fast as possible to prevent him from falling or injuring himself in any other way.

5. Go for help urgently, and move below any exposed ridge as soon as possible in case you are struck by the next flash.

MISCARRIAGE
SEE BLEEDING, page 77.

NOSEBLEED
SEE BLEEDING, page 74.

PERIOD PAINS

Before we explain about period pains, a warning about periods.

If you are a woman who suffers if she takes extra exercise during her periods, it is common sense not to go hill-walking or climbing at this time. If, also, you usually bleed heavily during your periods, you would be wise to avoid these activities then. You can more easily get fatigued, and a pleasurable day in the hills can turn into a tiring ordeal. So if you have, or are expecting, your period and suspect that it might affect your stamina, the best advice must be: Don't go out. Nor should any group insist on women or girls joining an outing if they have, or expect, a period.

What Are They?

Normally, the contractions of the womb as it sheds blood during a monthly period are so gentle that they cannot be felt. However, sometimes the contractions are more violent and cause painful spasms of the womb. The woman may double up or squirm with the pain, and she may also get backache. If the period is severe, its effect, and that of the pain, can be like a mild form of shock. The victim may feel hot and cold, may look pale and feel faint, and may even vomit.

What Can I Do?

First of all, relax and be patient. While this is not a medical emergency, the victim should never be put down as 'just hysterical'. Stop and let her rest in the position most comfortable to her. She may want to squat or curl up on the ground. If she wants to lie down, insulate the ground under her. A sterile dressing can be used as a sanitary towel. Comfort and reassure her: she may be embarrassed and upset that she is delaying the party, for period pains are usually a private affliction. Let her know that she is among friends – your positive attitude is important.

Eating and drinking may also help if the victim does not feel sick. However, there is no single remedy – a cup of hot sweet tea may help one woman, while making another quite sick. The victim may be carrying her usual remedy for period pains; or she, or you, may have some other pain-killing tablets.

The victim may feel much better within half an hour. If so, she should take the best route down with two other members of the group. Bad bouts of period pain can last up to three hours, some longer still. In this kind of situation, other factors, such as weather conditions and the amount of daylight left, will also have to be considered when you decide whether to send for help (see page 39).

SHOCK

Emergency Action Quick Reference

1. After any serious accident or illness, expect shock. Check that victim is still breathing and his heart is beating. If not, start artificial resuscitation (see page 54).
2. Don't move the victim unnecessarily.
3. Control external bleeding and watch for symptoms of internal bleeding.
4. Protect the victim from the cold, but do not overheat.
5. Keep him reassured and calm.
6. Go for help.

When we talk in everyday terms about somebody being shocked, we usually mean that they are extremely surprised, offended or amazed by the unexpected. There is little connection between this feeling of surprise and outrage and the complex body reaction which occurs after accident or injury, and which we also call shock. The latter is a physical condition which can kill a victim within minutes if unchecked. Few understand the real dangers of shock or how to control it.

A fatal accident is often accounted for by the explanation that the victim died of his injuries; while in fact, in many cases, he dies of shock long before he would die from the injuries themselves. Shock can be a fatal chain of events set in motion by even relatively minor accidents.

What Happens in Cases of Shock?

Shock is a failure in the blood-circulation system, caused when blood pressure drops too low to pump enough blood through the vital organs of the body and back to the heart. Although these organs could survive for a little while with an insufficient supply, the brain cannot manage without a constant adequate supply of the oxygen and other vital substances brought to it by the blood. Unless something can be done to correct the pressure, death will follow. Thus shock is the effect of the inadequate blood supply caused by sudden low pressure.

When Is It Likely to Occur?

It is fairly safe to assume that after any serious accident or attack of illness shock will develop, causing a problem additional to the injury or illness itself. To treat the injury, you will have to deal with shock; and by lessening the effects of shock, you will also reduce the damage being caused by the injury, the two being inseparable. However, in many cases of extreme injury, taking care of the shock first will save life.

One of the main causes of shock in mountain accidents is bleeding. With such rough and stony ground, a fall can result in deep cuts and open wounds, and the casualty often loses a large amount of blood in a short time. When there is less blood for the heart to pump round the body, the blood pressure drops quickly and shock follows.

However, obvious external bleeding is not the sole cause, or necessarily the prime cause, of shock. A victim suffering from internal injuries can be experiencing a very serious blood loss which may not be apparent if there are no outward signs.

In the case of burns, the blood vessels are damaged and leak plasma or fluid. There may be no external sign of this loss, but the body may react in the same way to the crisis of its reduced blood supply, by dropping pressure, causing shock. In addition, pain and mental anxiety can contribute considerably to the ill effects of shock.

Another common instance of shock follows the quite frequent incidents of heart attack, or coronary thrombosis, on the hills (see page 128). In this case, the heart muscle is damaged and cannot pump blood efficiently, and a sudden drop in blood pressure results in shock.

What Should I Notice?

The most obvious signs of shock are the actions that the body is already taking to compensate for its reduced flow of blood. When blood vessels narrow to restrict supply to non-essential parts of the body in order to keep the vital parts well supplied, the skin will look pale, and the victim feels cold and shivery, and may even break out in a cold sweat. The pulse may be either very slow or very rapid, and both abnormalities may indicate a state of shock.

What Can I Do?

1. Check immediately that the victim is breathing, and that his heart is beating. One of the first effects of severe shock may be failure of both, so be prepared to start artificial resuscitation at once (see page 54).

2. Don't move a badly injured person from the position in which he has fallen or collapsed unless his life is in immediate danger if he remains where he is. Victims of very serious injuries on the hills have actually been killed

by clumsy attempts to move them. This action may make injuries or bleeding worse, or cause more pain, and these factors can contribute even further to the already dangerously low blood pressure.

3. Control any blood loss to prevent a further drop in pressure, by exerting direct pressure over the wound using a sterile dressing and padding, as described on page 71.

4. Remain calm and reassuring. The importance of your own mental attitude towards the victim after an accident cannot be over-stressed in the control of shock. The victim's own distress may worsen the effects of shock, and you could contribute to this by transmitting your own anxieties to him. Let him feel that you are in charge of the situation, and give him confidence.

5. While the position of collapse on the ground may be the most natural for the body's own recovery mechanisms, the victim must still be protected from the cold. Cover him, but don't make him hot. Prevent him from shivering or becoming cold. In the past, stress has been placed on the importance of keeping an accident victim warm, but recently it has been discovered that in some cases this can have an adverse effect on his survival. If you warm him too much, blood will rush to the outer surface of the body, when it is needed to keep the inner parts supplied. However, while not over-heating, remember also that shock can make the casualty more susceptible to hypothermia.

6. Generally, it is wiser not to give the victim anything to eat in case there are internal injuries or damage to the digestive system.

Can I Give a Drink?

Yes. This could help to control shock, and the benefits will probably outweigh the risk of any damage you may cause internally. However, if shock is only part of a specific injury or illness, follow the direction on this point given in that section. NEVER give alcohol. The traditional practice of giving shocked people a measure of brandy is very dangerous because all alcohol automatically lowers blood pressure even further, increasing shock rather than reducing it.

Should I Send for Help?

Yes, even if the victim seems to be recovering.

SNAKE BITES

There are three types of snake in Britain: the grass snake, or ringed snake; the smooth snake; and the adder, or viper. By far the most common is the adder – in fact, no other snake is found in Scotland. The adder is the only one of the three with a poisonous bite. It can be found almost anywhere, but prefers open moorlands, sandy heaths and hillsides well exposed to the sun, although it is possible to find adders in any rough open country, including high ground. In Ireland there are no snakes at all.

Most people regard snake bites as a fatal calamity, but not all bites are serious, let alone deadly. Sometimes attempts at first aid prove more dangerous than the bite itself, with misguided heroes trying do-it-yourself surgery and other unnecessary panic measures. However, as you are just as likely, or unlikely, to be bitten by a snake in the Cairngorms as the New Forest, it is necessary to know the correct first aid in case medical treatment is not close at hand.

All snakes have small teeth, so it follows that all snakes can bite a victim, but only the bite of the adder presents any danger. British snakes are shy, timid creatures and are far more frightened of you than you could possibly be of them. The adder will attack only if it feels threatened, as can happen if you take it by surprise and step on it unawares, or if you try to catch it or pick it up, which it dislikes intensely. If it hears you coming, it will normally make off as fast as it can, but adders cannot move very quickly and may attack before moving if you are very close.

If you are not sure whether you are face to fang with an adder or a grass snake, remember that the adder has very distinctive markings, although no two are exactly the same. The hallmark of the adder is the telltale dark zigzag stripe which runs down the middle of its back, and it is thicker, heavier and shorter than the grass snake or smooth snake. A grass snake is olive brown, olive grey or olive green above, with black spots marking a pattern of vertical bars on its sides, and two rows of smaller spots, arranged alternately, on its back. The smooth snake looks more like an adder, but it is longer and has more polished scales, and if examined closely it can be seen that its pattern of spots on its back are really nothing like the adder's zigzags.

When Are They Most Likely to Occur?

Snakes hibernate in nests in winter, emerging in early spring on warm, sunny days. They enjoy basking in the sun in summer but they do not like strong heat, so the most likely time to find one at large at the height of a warm summer would probably be early morning. Although springtime is the commonest time to see adders, there is evidence that they sometimes hibernate in the roots of thick heather, so you may disturb a winter nest unwittingly in the hills, especially in Scotland.

What Happens When an Adder Bites?

The snake releases through its fang a substance called venom, which acts as a powerful depressant of the heart once it reaches the bloodstream. Venom is only harmful when it passes directly into the blood. It can be swallowed without danger as long as there are no sores or cuts in the mouth by which it could enter the blood. If a sufficiently large dose of venom is injected into the skin via the bite, death could follow rapidly from heart failure, and almost always does in the kind of small animals on which the snake preys for food. But the snake does not always give the maximum dose in a bite: his supply of venom may have been exhausted by previous recent use, or he may be inefficient at injecting the venom. The effect of a bite on the victim also varies considerably. Several factors are involved; one is the body weight of the victim. The bigger the person, the less harmful the bite is likely to be, which is why children suffer far more dramatically from the effects of venom than adults. The health of the bitten person also has some bearing on his resistance to the venom.

Very few people actually die from snake bites in Britain. Only ten deaths have been recorded during the last seventy years, and most of these were of children. But, nonetheless, these bites can make a victim very ill, although there are probably just as many cases of bites having little or no ill effects.

What Does It Look Like?

Typical places for bites are on the hands, feet, ankles and calves. Bites produce two different sets of symptoms. The first ill effects are felt in the bitten area, which starts to swell. Sometimes the swelling spreads further up the limb, and the skin may become discoloured. The second symptom varies from a mild feeling of sickness to complete collapse in a very short time. If the victim is very badly affected by the bite, he will vomit, have diarrhoea, feel giddy and eventually become unconscious, and he will also be suffering from shock. When the bite proves fatal, the victim gradually gets weaker, his pulse fades and he finds it increasingly hard to breathe. Death occurs any time between about six and sixty hours, caused by eventual heart failure.

What Can I Do?

1. The victim may be shocked, so check that breathing and heart beat have not been affected. If they have, artificial resuscitation may be necessary should either fail (see page 54). Treat for shock (page 153).

2. Antidotes, in the form of drugs or serum, are required, and if the effects of the bite become serious send for help urgently.

3. Keep the victim as still as possible to slow down the rate at which the venom is being absorbed into the bloodstream. Immobilization of the affected limb as in the case of fracture may further slow down the process.

4. Remain alert in case breathing difficulty occurs.

5. In the case of only minor ill effects from venom, it may be possible to help the victim to make his own way down to safety, but watch for any signs of deterioration in his condition.

What Not to Do

Three first-aid methods, which are widely thought to be useful for snake bites, often cause more damage than the bite itself. These rather drastic and dramatic measures probably date back to Colonial times when many British subjects saw at first hand the horrifying effects of the highly poisonous snakes of India and elsewhere, which can kill within minutes. Such methods are not necessary to counteract adder venom. So:

1. DON'T use a tourniquet to try to prevent the venom from circulating in the bloodstream. The tourniquet is a dangerous first-aid technique which could eventually cost the victim a limb, if the circulation is restricted for long enough. No victim of an adder bite would thank you if he recovered naturally from a moderately serious bite, only to lose his arm or leg unnecessarily.

2. DON'T cut open the bite to release the venom by sucking it out. This extreme first aid may be justified in the case of a highly venomous tropical snake bite, but it has no place on the hills of Britain. To do such a thing would involve a high risk of infection, as well as increasing the effects of shock and causing bleeding.

3. DON'T give alcohol; this can speed up the absorption of the venom.

Victims of adder bites may seem unaffected by the attack, but it is still necessary to keep a careful watch for several hours in case the venom is slow acting.

You can avoid snake bites by leaving peace-loving adders well alone, and by treating all snakes in Britain as though they were adders if you cannot distinguish them. Do not handle snakes, and protect feet and legs in known snake habitations by wearing thick-soled boots, and trousers tucked into thick socks, leaving no skin exposed.

SNOWBLINDNESS

If you have ever walked or climbed in a country which has a climate combining snow and sunshine in very dry, cold conditions, you will be aware of the dangers of snowblindness and you will have noticed everybody wearing goggles or dark glasses to protect their eyes.

In Ireland and the lowlands of Britain, winter temperatures are not normally low enough to prevent snow melting in sunshine, but on the hills, and especially in Scotland, snow conditions like those in the Alps are fairly common in winter. Mild cases of snowblindness occur occasionally when walkers and climbers are unaware of the dangers of snow and sunshine together.

What Is It?

Snowblindness is not just the white glare which we experience when sunlight is reflected by snow. If we look for long enough, the cornea of the eye is actually burnt by the reflected ultra-violet rays of the sun, and this results in very intense pain and swelling. Although there is very little first aid that you can do to help the victim of snowblindness, you can at least be forewarned and take the right precautions. If it does occur, you can also prevent it from getting worse.

When Is It Likely to Happen?

Snowblindness occurs in dry, sunny, frosty weather following a snowfall, if the victim faces the glare of the snow as he walks or climbs without eye protection. The higher the altitude, the greater the risk.

What Can I Do?

1. There is nothing you can do to ease the pain until you reach safety, and the condition can be treated by a doctor.

2. However, you can make the victim more comfortable by the use of dark glasses if available, or makeshift goggles made of cardboard, for example, out of a food packet. Using scissors from the first-aid kit, cut two narrow horizontal slits so that the eyes are protected but the victim can see where he is going. You can keep the improvised goggles on by tucking each end of the cardboard inside the victim's anorak hood or hat by the side of his face. As soon as it is practical, cover the eyes either with pads or bandages until you get medical help.

SPINAL INJURIES

Emergency Action Quick Reference

1. Check that any spinal injury has not paralysed muscles in the neck affecting breathing, and ensure that the airway remains unobstructed in an unconscious victim. Start artificial respiration if breathing fails (see page 54).

2. If the victim complains of numbness, loss of movement or paralysis in any part of his body after a fall involving his back, don't move him unless his life is in danger.

3. Call for help urgently, protect him from the cold, and leave him lying face downwards if possible.

Spinal injuries are extremely serious in themselves but can easily be made worse or fatal by the slightest move in the wrong direction. The spinal cord is the vital link which controls the relaying of messages between the brain and the rest of the body. In many cases of spinal damage, the protective bones, called the vertebrae, through which the spinal cord is threaded are fractured, and the movement of these broken bones can cause pinching, bruising or more serious damage including severing of the cord. In general, the higher up the cord that the damage is done, the larger the extent of the body affected. If an injury occurs at the top of the spine, it may affect breathing by paralysis of the neck muscles as well as causing loss of feeling and movement everywhere else in the body below the injury. The two greatest dangers of spinal injury are a failure of breathing through paralysis; and permanent paralysis of various parts of the body should the fragments of broken vertebrae cut across the cord, destroying its capacity to carry messages from the brain.

When Should I Suspect a Spinal Injury?

After any heavy or long fall involving the neck, or back, be most careful to examine the victim for spinal injury and treat him accordingly even if you are uncertain if damage has occurred. Several important signs may indicate the seriousness of the injury. Look for any paralysis or loss of feeling in any part of the body; any tingling sensation or numbness; inability to control the bladder and bowels; or severe pain in the back and neck. These signs can warn you of the gravity of the injury if there are no other visible signs of spinal damage except bruising or swelling.

What Can I Do?

1. If the victim is unconscious, check that he can breathe without difficulty. If the neck muscles become paralysed by the injury, start mouth-to-mouth assisted breathing (see

page 59). This will have to continue until the victim reaches hospital and a machine can be used, so others will have to be ready to take over the assisted breathing and share the task. In this condition, however, the victim may not survive.

2. If the victim is conscious, keep a check on his breathing in case his neck muscles become paralysed, and ask him to describe areas of pain or loss of sensation. If he tells you he cannot move any part of his body, or if you notice that he cannot control his bladder, spinal injury is very likely and you must not move him unless he is in danger of further injury by staying where he has fallen. If he is lying on his face, leave him as he is. If he is lying on his back, gently place padding under each side of the injured part, but do not do this if it is necessary to move him.

3. Send for help urgently, telling whoever goes to make sure that rescuers know a spinal injury is likely. Some teams are equipped with special spinal splints and stretchers.

4. If you have to move the victim to save his life, do it preferably with four people lifting him horizontally, as if he were rigid, avoiding any spinal movement.

5. Protect both the conscious and the unconscious victim from the cold while waiting for help, and do nothing more than the essentials of resuscitation if necessary, and control of any bleeding.

STINGS
SEE INSECT STINGS, pages 144–8.

SUNSTROKE
SEE HEATSTROKE, pages 131–4.

VARICOSE VEINS
SEE BLEEDING, pages 76–7.

VERTIGO

Vertigo is a widely used term, and it can mean anything from a disorder of balance-control in the ear, which gives the impression that surrounding objects are moving when they are not, to dizziness or a desperate fear of heights or of falling. Although there are certain physical causes of such giddiness, when vertigo occurs on the hills it is usually because the victim is afraid and it is caused by a state of mind as much as of body.

Often, people who are afraid of heights know about their fear before they start to climb or walk in steep places. Many of them avoid hills for this reason, while some of them attempt walking and climbing in order to help overcome the fear. But the danger really lies when the victim develops this fear unexpectedly while he is on the hills. Unless help is given rapidly, it has been known for victims to become hysterical and even to cause the deaths of fellow climbers by their uncontrolled fear.

Vertigo of this sort, with its basis in fear, or insecurity, may not be noticed when the beginner does his first easy climbs. These climbs usually have plenty of holds and ledges to break up the steepness of the face, so the novice does not encounter any feeling of insecurity. However, on his first difficult climb he may become aware, especially on a very smooth rock face, of a feeling of 'exposure', which is how experienced climbers describe the insecurity of realizing that there is very little to break a fall between themselves and the ground. This feeling can also occur when walkers are scrambling over rough ground.

What Happens to a Victim Suffering from Vertigo?

The victim's first reaction is usually 'I can't go on', and he may quickly become very distressed, and start to sweat, or cry, or shout, and his fears will become more and more extreme and his behaviour more unreasonable.

What Can I Do?

1. Reassure the victim. This is the most important first aid before anything else, so that the victim will not endanger his own and other people's lives with his growing fear. Each situation will be different, but as a general rule it may not help much to adopt the 'pull yourself together' attitude. Climbing instructors treat vertigo very seriously, and many of them say that the first step in helping the victim is confident but kindly and firm reassurance, without anger at the victim who is putting others at risk.

2. Once you have reassured the victim that he is in no danger and is able to cope with the problem, or the next move, concentrate on getting him down as soon as possible. Don't force him to continue, in the hope that he can overcome his fear. It may recur, and his mood and actions might be quite unpredictable.

3. Some climbers have their own patent ways of dealing with vertigo, for instance by making the victim focus on an object which breaks up the sensation of sheer drop underneath him. If you have any ideas like this, they could be valuable as long as you have faith in them, and the victim has faith in you and your capabilities to help him. Whatever the notion, the aim is simply to calm the victim down sufficiently to get him to help himself down to safety.

BIBLIOGRAPHY

AIR FORCE DEPARTMENT: *Mountain Rescue*, H.M.S.O., 1972.

BLACKSHAW, ALAN: *Mountaineering: From Hill-Walking to Alpine Climbing*, Penguin Books, 1970.

CLARKE, CHARLES, WARD, MICHAEL, and WILLIAMS, EDWARD (eds.): *Mountain Medicine and Physiology*, The Alpine Club, 1975.

CREW, PETER: *Encyclopaedic Dictionary of Mountaineering*, Constable, 1968.

DISLEY, JOHN: *Orienteering*, Faber, 1969.

First Aid Manual, British Red Cross, St Andrew's Ambulance Association and St John Ambulance Brigade, 1972.

GREENBANK, ANTHONY: *Survival for Young People*, Harrap, 1975.

JACKSON, JOHN: *Safety on Mountains*, British Mountaineering Council, 1975.

LANGMUIR, ERIC: *Mountain Leadership*, Scottish Sports Council, 1969.

MACINNES, HAMISH: *International Mountain Rescue Handbook*, Constable, 1972.

Map Reading, Know the Game Series, Educational Productions, 1965.

Mountain Rescue and Cave Rescue, Mountain Rescue Committee, annually.

PAULCKE, WILHELM, and DUMLER, HELMUT: *Hazards in Mountaineering*, Kaye & Ward, 1973.

STEELE, PETER: *Medical Care for Mountain Climbers*, Heinemann Medical Books, 1976.

SUTTON, O. G.: *Understanding Weather*, Penguin Books, 1960.

UNSWORTH, WALT: *Encyclopaedia of Mountaineering*, Robert Hale, 1975; Penguin Books, 1977.

Printed by
Carnmor Print & Design
95/97 London Road, Preston.